Books For Reading On Line. Com

Books That Make A Difference

We support diabetes research and other charitable and research organisations.
10% of all books sold is donated to these charities

ISBN: 978-0-6481884-2-1

Copyright© 2018 MSI Australia
All rights reserved.

Published by Books For Reading On Line.Com
Company Registration No: 642 923 859

Under license from MSI Ltd, Australia
NSW, Australia

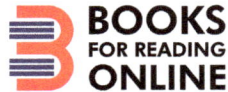

BOOKS
FOR READING
ONLINE

See our website: www.booksforreadingonline.com

Or contact by email: sales@booksforreadingonline.com or: admin@booksforreadingonline.com

Front & Back Covers and Copyright owned by MSI, Australia

MSI acknowledges the author of the images used in this book.

Photography and illustrations by Christine Thompson-Wells ©

Contents   Page

For You – The Beginning Of An Extraordinary Journey...

Life is full of surprises. A greater surprise can come about when you discover your own inner strength and tenacity. By stopping, listening to your inner voice, and taking the time to respect the great internal gifts you have, life's journey can become an exciting adventure.

As you read and work through the different essential flower and plant oils, you will discover the awakening of your senses; the power the oil contains, and how this power can transcend within you and work with your higher self.

Included in the book are the steps to take in learning how to breathe properly. Breathing correctly is essential to maintaining good health and wellbeing. By breathing properly essential oils can add to your quality of life, happiness, and longevity.

It's the combination of breathing properly and using essential oils, I believe, that will allow the human being, regardless of any situation, to become grounded, responsible and work through the most difficult of experiences.

Stress is inevitable in life, in fact, if we did not have stress in our lives, we would never get any jobs done, bills paid, or other mundane tasks accomplished. It's too much of the wrong type of stress that causes pain, illness, heart attacks and disease. By working with your breathing on a daily basis, using essential oils as though they were your best friend and understanding how your human system, including your mind works, your life gains a quality of wellbeing that may have eluded you over your life time.

Not all oils are for all people; there is a certain resonance about an oil that works with you. You will feel comfortable, at ease, satisfied and know that you are working with a unique combination. As you work through your life and life experiences, you will understand that each oil essence is different – oils will fit different situations and conditions.

Over time, your needs and demands will change – an essential oil you once loved may become redundant; this is not the fault of the oil; you have changed and the conditions you are working with may have changed. There are different oils for different human experiences.

Having said, all of the above, it's important to breathe properly – it's the combination of breathing and enjoying essential oils that will make the difference in your life.

Inspiration

When I write a book it's because I have had an inner calling from either my mind or a message from my inner voice that speaks loudly and says: 'start writing' and then the topic is made clear as the words appear on the page.

My writings are varied from poetry, to how to work with cash flow, mind health, managing stress and 'how to' books on creating flower arrangements; I also write children's books including adventure stories and other genre that I am guided to write.

Having received one of these messages, I was in the finishing stages of writing, taking the photographs and drawing the diagrams for How To Create Easy Wedding Bouquets when I was told: 'that now needs to be done...' referring to this latest book: Healing & Wellbeing from Flowers & Plants – making the most of the power of essential oils.

There is no doubt, I enjoy a challenge and this latest book, though I have always had a fascination for the energy and power of flowers and plants, was a challenge – it has been a most satisfying and enjoyable journey.

The contents of the book were up to me; I have relied on my inspiration and the positive universal energy sent forth. I must admit, I do ask for guidance and help continually – to me, it's the only way the books can be created.

I consider myself to be an instrument and the flow of energy connected to the words which appear on the paper are directed from somewhere other than from my own source of inspiration. Having said that, I think many writers feel this same way…

Essential Oil Droplets

Each essential oil is basically made up of minute-droplets. These droplets are transported from the senses by the motor neuron pathways that run throughout the human body. The human nose is responsible for part of the transporting of the scent of the essential oil. On reaching the brain, the limbic system takes over. The limbic system is a set of brain structures, including your smelling capacity (olfactory) and other sensory responses. Included within this system is your capacity for emotional response, motivation to be active and do something, long-term memory, and your thought processes.

The essence from the droplets that are inhaled will enter your body's circulatory system, will reach your lungs, from this point they will disperse throughout your body. This is the power of essential oil.

Essential Oils and Their Healing Power

Many of us go through life and don't understand the power of the flowers and plants around us. It is now time to open-up the windows, doorways, and the human mind to welcome into, not only my life, but the lives of the readers I write so many books for.

Having trained as a florist so many years ago; the different flowers and plants that grow on this wonderful Planet of ours never ceases to amaze me. Plants and flowers grow from the wilderness of Patagonia, to the Arctic Circle and the Sahara Desert; each contributing to the health and wellbeing of this Planet we call home. Having said the above, many of us still struggle to see these treasures of nature as we live our daily lives.

Just by looking at a flower or plant can bring healing into people's lives. Often, it's taking the time to **just stop**, look and take in the beauty for this healing process to begin.

Many people are familiar with essential oils and some of their healing values. I'm going to go a little deeper to look at how these essential oils hold the power to effectively give us healing.

On the opposite page and on page (2), I have given five lists of essential oils I am going speak about. Each oil is unique, each holds within its essence the power to heal and bring about wellbeing. Essential oils are a gift from nature each has properties that provide healing for human beings, animals, and insects. Not only can these oils help to renew the human body, but they work with the human mind to rebalance and soothe many disorders both mental and physical leading to overall personal wellbeing

Wellbeing leads to life satisfaction, personal positive-growth, and the fulfilment of dreams.

Essential Oils

Important Essential Oils

Perfume Oils ~ FLOWERS

GERANIUM
BERGAMOT
ATTAR OF ROSES
YLANG-YLANG
TUBEROSE
PATCHOULI
JASMINE
SCENTED BORONIA
LAVENDER
GARDENIA
IMMORTELLE

Essential Oils

Important Essential Oils

Perfume Oils ~ GRASSES

CITRONELLA
LEMON GRASS
VETIVER

Essential Oils

Important Essential Oils

Wood Oils

CADE
CAMPHOR
CEDARWOOD
EUCALYPTUS
SANDALWOOD
SASSAFRAS
PINE NEEDLES
CINNAMON

Essential Oils

Important Essential Oils

Herb Oils

BASIL
CORIANDER
OREGANO
ROSEMARY
PARSLEY
CHAMOMILE
HOPS

Essential Oils

Important Essential Oils

Flavouring Oils

PEPPERMINT
SPEARMINT
STAR ANISE
CELERY
CLOVES
LEMON
ORANGE
LIME
CARAWAY
NUTMEG
THYME

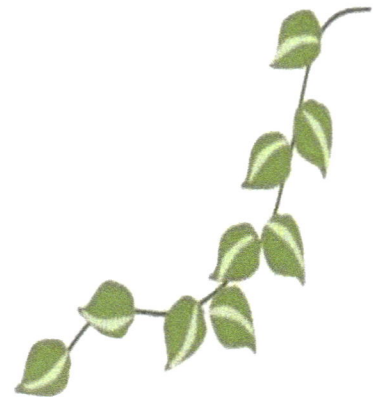

Flower Oils ~ Healing & Wellbeing from Essential Oils

Flower Oils and Their Healing Power

GERANIUM

This delicate flower and its extracted essential oil hold many health benefits as a treatment in aromatherapy. It has the ability, to uplift the human spirit, improve mental wellbeing and add to emotional balance.

Other health benefits include:

- ❖ Reduce stress
- ❖ Balance hormones
- ❖ Reduce inflammation
- ❖ Improve circulation
- ❖ Reduce blood pressure
- ❖ Reduce depression
- ❖ Reduce the effects of menopause
- ❖ Improve dental health
- ❖ Help to repair skin scar tissue.

Citronella or lemon scented leaf geraniums release a scent when they are touched; touching the leaves may have other benefits to the human mind and body incorporating the human psyche.

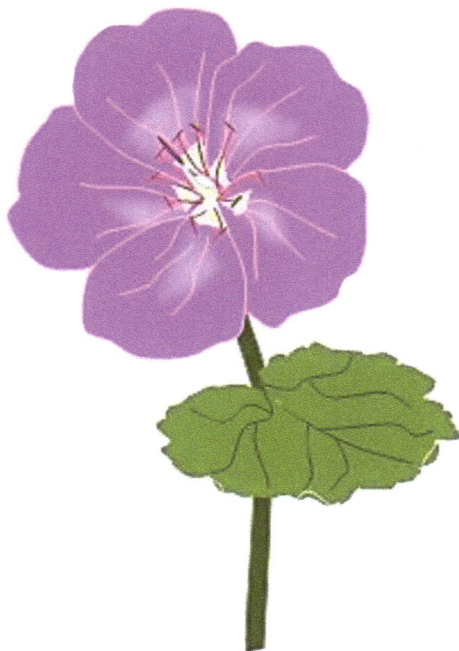

Scents such as lemon and citronella act on our sense of smell and through the transition from the touch, which releases the essential oil, this travels to your nostrils' thus the information, through neuron receptors, is transported to the brain. Good smells and experiences help to develop good physical health, good mind health and wellbeing.

This ancient oil was used by the Egyptians to promote healthy and radiant skin.

BERGAMOT

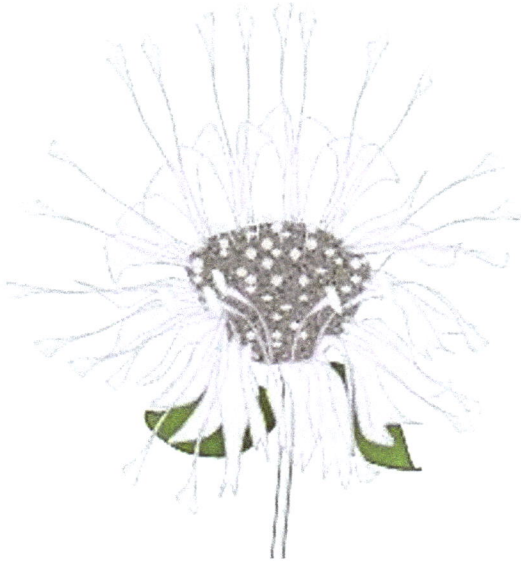

Bergamot is related to the citrus family and is used to:

- ❖ Relax nervous tension
- ❖ Reduce stress
- ❖ Can be used as a sedative
- ❖ Reduce anxiety
- ❖ Helps to reduce high blood pressure
- ❖ Helps in sleep disorders
- ❖ Assist in reducing depression
- ❖ Helps with cleansing the skin.

Bergamot can be made into a tea which helps to produce calming at stressful times.

Bergamot will assist with some skin disorders such as acne. For teenagers, it helps to unclog pores in pimple breakouts and will help to rebalance oily skin.

Bergamot can easily blend with other essential oils.

In mythological stories, bergamot is associated with the sun and has been used in rituals to clear the mind, lighten the spirit and effective in managing some areas of depression. Bergamot is associated with spiritual rebalance that allows us to reconnect with our higher self and our positive energy input.

Connecting with higher energy allows us to unlock our creativity, focus on the 'here and now' and allows us to find more easily the happiness and humour that's in life's trivial events.

ATTAR OF ROSES

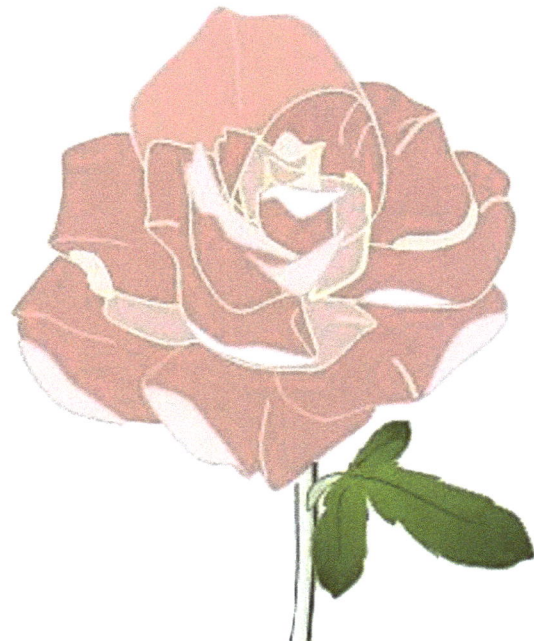

Roses have been used for thousands of years for medicinal purposes. Ironically, it wasn't until the 19th Century that rose petals were distilled in water and the oil used in aromatherapy.

Essential rose oil or rose tea can be used to:

- ❖ Relieve stress
- ❖ Reduce depression
- ❖ Reduce sinus congestion
- ❖ Alleviate cold symptoms
- ❖ Help with digestive ailments
- ❖ Assist with healing sore throats
- ❖ Help to reduce nausea

- ❖ Assist with reducing coughing
- ❖ Help with menopausal symptoms or disorder
- ❖ Assist with sleep disorders.

Rose hips have been valued as a food; in 1934 were identified as the richest source of vitamin C.

The scent of rose oil, when rubbed externally, is very soothing for the nervous system and promotes calmness within the human system.

*The Attar of rose is the scent obtained from the distillation of the oil from the Damask rose.

YLANG YLANG

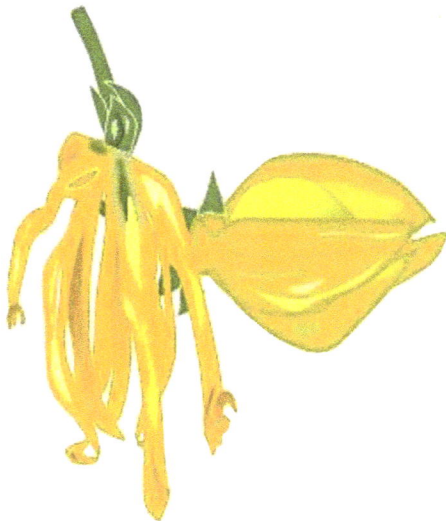

The use of ylang-ylang as a medicinal has come down to us over many hundreds of years. In Edwardian and Victorian times, ylang-ylang oil was mixed with coconut oil to create Macassar hair oil used by both men and women. The oil helped to promote shine and to keep it in place.

Ylang-ylang can be used to:

- ❖ Help to reduce depression
- ❖ Promote relaxation
- ❖ Assist with insomnia

- ❖ Reduce blood pressure
- ❖ Assist as an antibacterial
- ❖ Increase sexual desire
- ❖ Helps to kill head lice.

Ylang-ylang is often used in aromatherapy or mixed with other essential oils which can make a very pleasant and effective massage oil.

The dried flowers of ylang-ylang can be used to lie between clothing or linen when stored over a period of time.

TUBEROSE

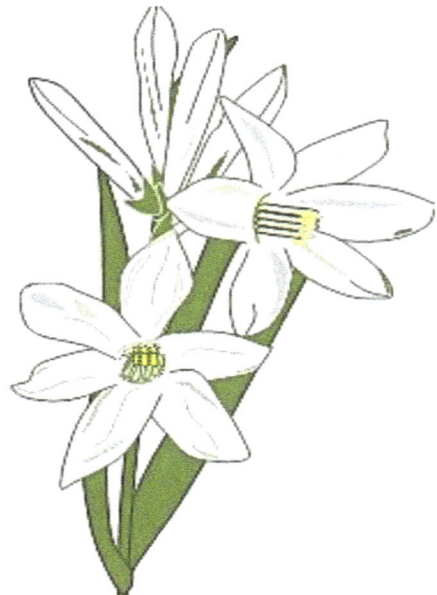

Tuberose is unknown in the wild but grows well in Central America and India. The flower gives off its intoxicating scent during evening and night. For perfume production, tuberose is grown in France and is a cultivated for its essential oil. Tuberose is known as the 'Night Queen' or 'Mistress of the Night'.

Tuberose can stimulate those parts of the brain to do with sensual pleasure, sexual feelings and raising libido. Tuberose has significant benefits to:

- ❖ Raise sexual arousal as an aphrodisiac
- ❖ Relieves stress and anxiety
- ❖ Increases blood circulation
- ❖ Eliminates bad odours
- ❖ When used in aromatherapy, the scent creates relaxation and may be used as a sedative.

The flowers leave a warm and inviting feeling when left in a vase in a room.

Because of their intoxicating scent, the tuberose has been used by florists' when they are creating wedding bouquets, decorating churches or in headdress designs when floral crowns are worn.

PATCHOULI

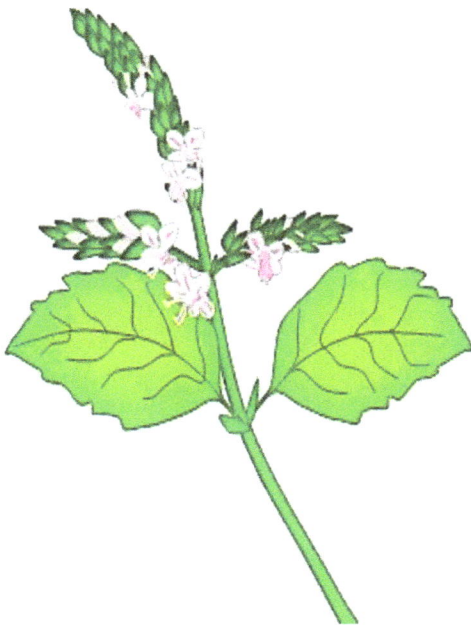

The leaves and young shoots of patchouli, when distilled, yield an oil which is used in aromatherapy and in other essential oils.

Patchouli has a warm, spicy, almost musky scent. It belongs to the family of mint, sage and lavender. Patchouli was known and is known as the scent of the sixties. Patchouli, at one time, was valued as highly as gold. One pound of patchouli was considered to be worth one pound of gold.

The health benefits of patchouli are:

- ❖ Assists with fighting depression
- ❖ Can assist as an antiseptic
- ❖ Assists with sleep disorders
- ❖ May be used as an aphrodisiac
- ❖ Has anti-fungal properties
- ❖ Assists with reducing stress and fatigue
- ❖ Helps with reducing headaches and head pain
- ❖ Assists with stabilising emotions for adults and children
- ❖ Can support emotional stability in times of severe stress.

When patchouli oil is added to massage oils it has grounding properties that support wellbeing of the mind allowing the body to re-balance.

When applied regularly to the skin, patchouli essential oil aids in reducing lines and blemishes and allows the skin to glow and appear radiant.

Other benefits of the oil, when a headache strikes: blend with a carrier oil, shake a few drops of the mixture onto a tissue and dab onto the temples and back of the neck.

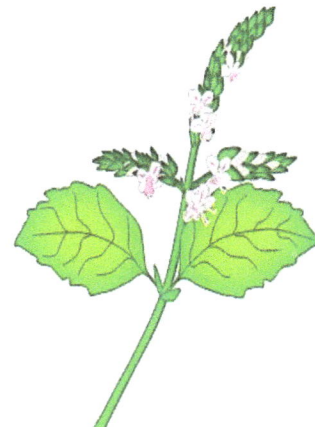

JASMINE

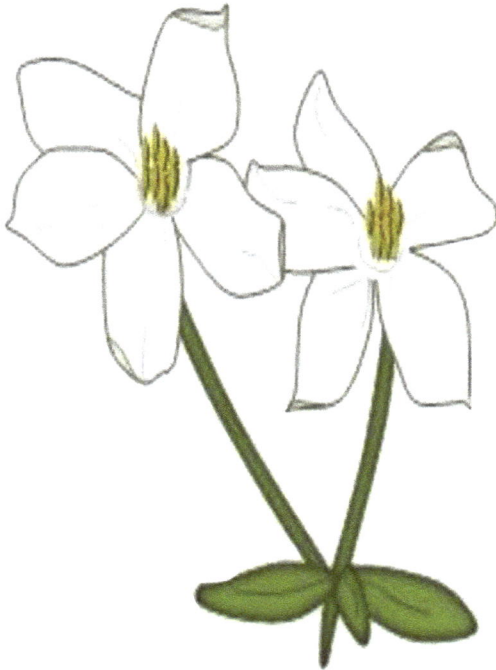

There are a number of different jasmine plants that grow throughout the world. The flowers of the plant *J. officinale* are used to make essential oils. These plants originated in the Himalayas.

The scent of jasmine is exotic and considered as a sacred flower throughout India and the Himalayas. Jasmine is also considered the flower of love.

Jasmine oil is said to be both mystical and spiritual in its healing properties.

In meditation, the use of jasmine oil is said to re-balance the body's chakras, by doing this, the facilitation of the third eye – the eye in the middle of the frontal lobe in the forehead – is awakened. This awakening engages people to connect with their:

- ❖ Wisdom
- ❖ Imagination
- ❖ Creativity and
- ❖ Clairvoyance

Other healing benefits from using jasmine essential oils include:

- ❖ Boosts and reduces mood swings
- ❖ Inhalation of the scent reduces phlegm
- ❖ Balances hormones and in women, helps in regulation of periods
- ❖ If you are breast feeding, it benefits in the flow of milk reducing the possibility of congested milk ducts
- ❖ In childbirth, jasmine assists with calming the mother and easing the pain of delivery
- ❖ Jasmine essential oil is said to lift the libido and stimulates arousal leading to romance and love.

Like all essential oils, some you will like and others not so. It may be a *try and see* and what works for you.

Seek medical or professional advice if you are pregnant or about to give birth – some oils are not recommended at these times.

SCENTED BORONIA

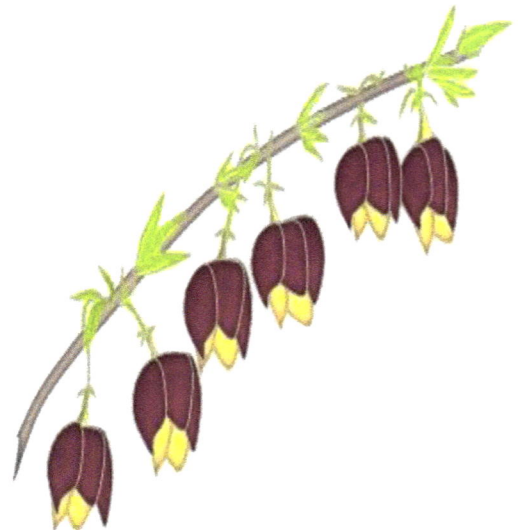

Boronias are native to Australia and the island of Tasmania; it is widely known as Cornish Pepper.

Brown boronia has a distinctive and intoxicating scent and once experienced, it's very difficult to not go back for more...

The flowers are beautifully shaped with a reddish-brown outer petal, later revealing a golden to yellow inside of the under petals.

Boronia essential oils are expensive to produce but are used in some aromatherapy. Boronia may assist in:

- ❖ Reducing stress and anxiety
- ❖ Help to overcome some emotional tension
- ❖ Assist with mood swings and re-stabilise emotions
- ❖ May be used to calm the mind
- ❖ The scent is fresh, uplifting and allows the human psyche to re-energise
- ❖ It may assist with helping to restore metabolic conditions such as an underactive thyroid
- ❖ Is an aphrodisiac and assists in restoring sexual drive and enjoyment.

Boronia is a rare oil because of the difficulties in growing the plant, therefore, oil production is uncommon. The power of the scent has left some to say: *'it's as close to heaven as you can get.'*

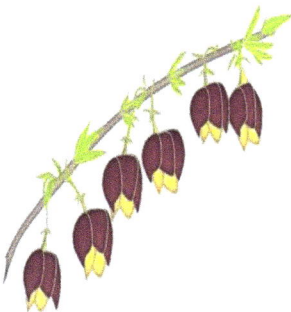

LAVENDER

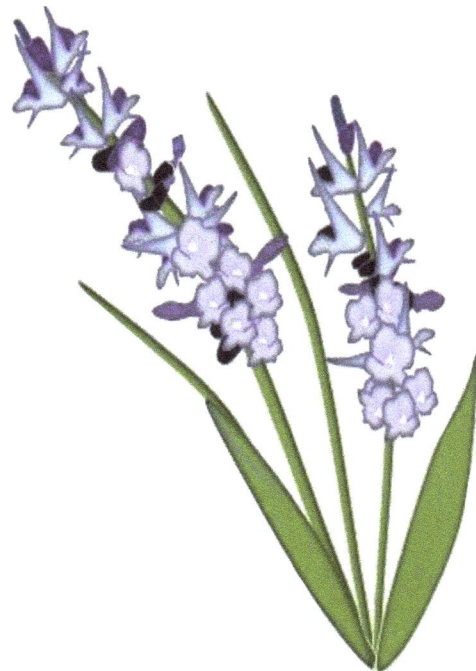

Like so many of the scented plants, lavender has its favourites. Lavender has been used for centuries for healing and wellbeing. It is however, *L. stoechas,* the variety of lavender that has been used since classical times as a medicinal preparation.

Pure lavender oil is obtained from *L. latifolia*.

Lavender oil has effective healing properties which have been used for over 3,000 years. It was used in Egypt for mummification of the dead and for healing many skin disorders.

In the 21st Century lavender oil is used in aromatherapy to aid with:

- ❖ Insomnia, thus, improves cognitive function
- ❖ Anxiety and stress
- ❖ Migraines, headaches, and depression
- ❖ Helps to regulate heart-rate variability
- ❖ Acne or skin breakouts

- ❖ Respiratory problems from colds and flu
- ❖ Backache and lumbago or lower back pain
- ❖ Lavender oil may assist with relieving asthma, bronchitis, whooping cough, laryngitis, and tonsillitis
- ❖ It helps with the circulation of blood through the body resulting in lower blood pressure and reduces hypertension
- ❖ It can be an effective treatment with psoriasis, burns and sunburns.

Lavender essential oil may be beneficial in helping to reduce weight – the scent assists with the gratification process connected to the brain's pleasure centre (ventral tegmental) area. Instead of wanting to eat a sweet biscuit, inhale a little lavender oil to satisfy your desires – it may just work for you.

Lavender oil has many benefits but like so many of the oils used in healing, it needs to be used in moderation.
Lavender oil blends with sage, geranium, pine, nutmeg, cedarwood and jasmine.

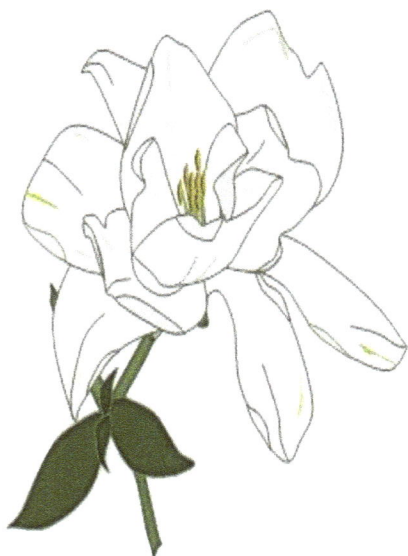

GARDENIA

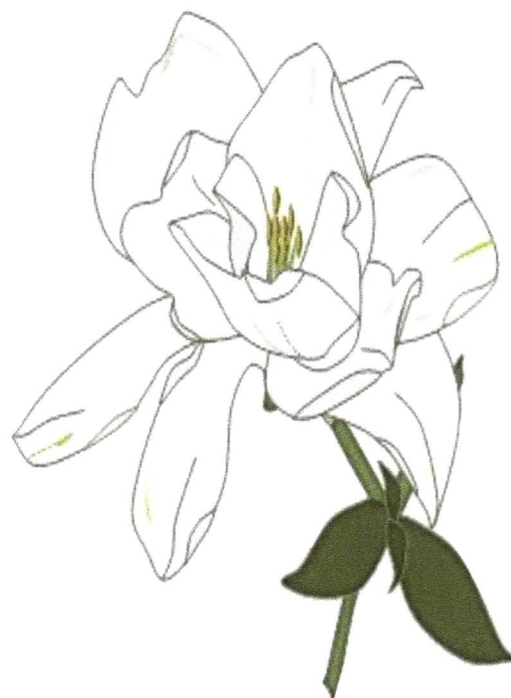

The beautiful fragrance of gardenia allows the mind to take a short holiday. Inhaling the scent can be intoxicating but the intoxication is worth every moment spent while one looks at the wonder of such beauty.

Surprisingly, the gardenia plant is related to the coffee family. The plant grows well in Australia, the tropical and sub-tropical regions of Asia, Africa, Madagascar, and the Pacific Islands.

Gardenia essential oil has beneficial values in treating:

- ❖ Anxiety
- ❖ Infections
- ❖ Menopausal imbalances and is good for cooling the blood
- ❖ Can be used as a sedative
- ❖ Helps to sooth headaches and migraine
- ❖ Assists with bladder infections
- ❖ Helps to heal skin disorders
- ❖ Releases nervous tension
- ❖ Helps to sooth sinus infections

- Is effective as an antibacterial and
- Helps to reduce swelling
- Assists with improving the libido in both men and women.

Essential oils have many properties that contain healing power; part of the process for any healing to take place is to believe: *plants contain unique qualities and hold a source of energy*. Because the power isn't seen by the naked eye, does not mean it doesn't exist!

Many professional people suggest to not use gardenia essential oil on pregnant woman or children.

IMMORTELLE

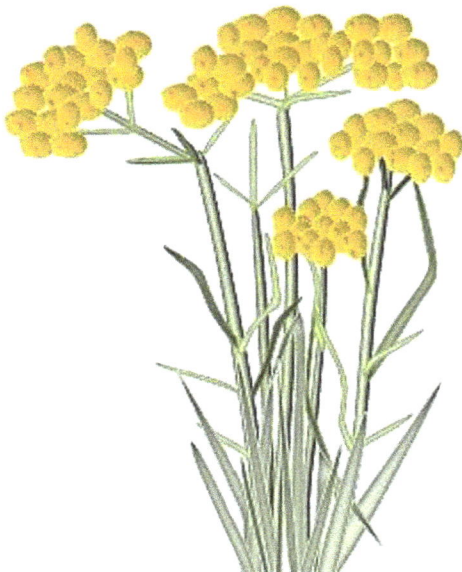

The immortelle flower and plant is known, not only for the precious oil it holds, but for the spiritual benefits it gives when used in aromatherapy and other meditative healing.

This delicate oil has regenerative properties for the skin; it is an anti-inflammatory and has proposed anti-cancer properties.

Other benefits of this oil when used in aromatherapy include:

- Releasing daily stressors and anxiety
- Helps in the release of emotional trauma
- In the spiritual sphere, it facilitates the connections to new positive experiences
- It develops stillness, peace and tranquillity while allowing the mind to rebalance
- Allows the mind to connect to the higher self-validating self-worth and positive growth
- When your skin suffers through sickness or accident, it will bring about inner wellbeing and skin to rejuvenation
- When used in massage, will help to alleviate joint and muscle pain
- For inhalation use 4-6 drops in a bowl of steaming water, not boiling, this helps to clear sinuses and helps to still the mind
- Will support the cardiovascular system by promoting blood flow
- Will assist in thinning blood and can be used as an anti-coagulant reducing haemorrhage
- Supports the immune system when it is under attack from colds and flu.

Immortelle oil is distilled from the stem of the plant. This is a soft, soothing oil, it blends well with rose, sage, lavender and citrus oils.

This particular oil offers many benefits for the heart, mind and soul while its regenerative properties are clearly seen when applied to the skin. When used in aromatherapy the essence and aroma go deeply into the human psyche allowing healing from past hurts and pain to work and restore positive mind health.

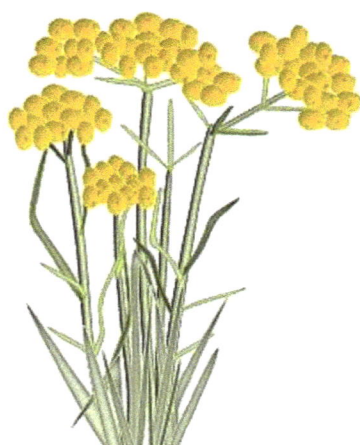

It's time to take a break.....

Learning How to Breathe

I believe flowers and essential oils have a form of positive energy – it's not seen, it cannot be touched, and the energy is only available, when we are ready to receive it. To be ready means: being ready in heart and mind and being in control of how we respond to this divine gift. One way I have found, is learning how to breathe correctly so that all of my energy is focused on the gift I am about to receive.

On the following page, I have outlined my breathing technique; I speak of and use this technique in my poem recordings within my Whispering Poem books. I have also run workshops using this same technique – the responses are remarkable. Please take just five minutes to enjoy your own discovery…

Breathing – The Joy

By doing the simple breathing exercise described below, you are creating a simple breathing feedback loop that works with you allowing you to relax, or, if you are experiencing stressful or difficult situations, it supports you to cope.

By breathing properly, the essential oils you use will interact with your bodily systems to support the healing you are doing. Breathing as described will aid the chakras to line up and the facilitation of the third eye – the eye in the middle of the frontal lobe in the forehead; this eye will awaken allowing for peace, creativity and wisdom to transpire.

To Begin:

1. Make sure your jaw is relaxed – unclench your jaw right now and feel the difference
2. Your feet and legs are uncrossed
3. Your shoulders are loose and not tense.

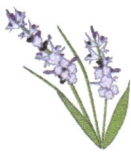

Breathe in through your nose – hold: count to 3

Push the air down into your lungs – hold: count to 3

Exhale the stale air through your mouth – hold: count of three – then start the process again.

Once you understand how to breathe, you can do it at any time and in any place.

Chakras are discrete energy centres that start at the top of the head and end at the bottom of the spine. They interact with all parts of the bodily system, affecting everything from resistance to disease to emotional processing.

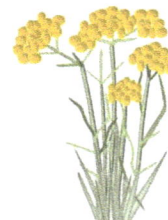

A Poem ~

Flowers

Flowers – these flowers we use
have taken millions of years to defuse...

They bring their healing power, their joy, their
forever love...

For their fascination they hold as their petals
unfold...

A gift of nature we see as we look – this magic
before us could not be written in any a book...

The essence extracted – the scent contained

A feeling of pleasure as the oil touches
your skin ~
this loving elixir helps healing begin...

The moments of pleasure as the perfume seeps
in...

Flowers ~ for their beauty within...

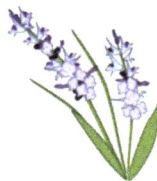

Grass Oils ~ Healing & Wellbeing from Essential Oils

Grass Oils and Their Healing Power

CITRONELLA

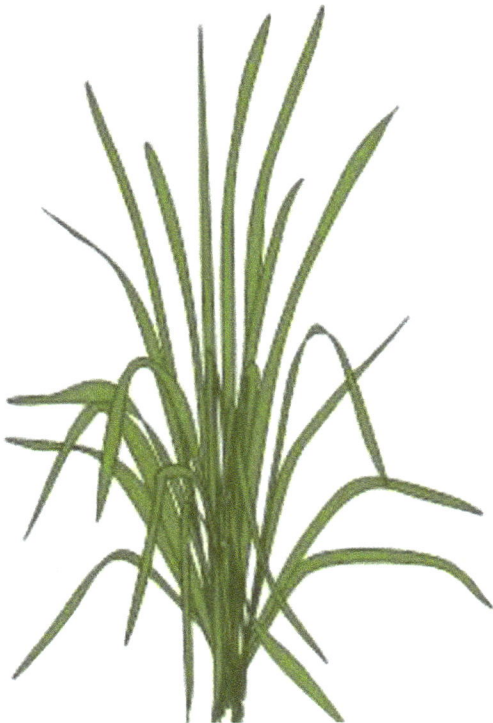

Citronella is found in many plants including mint, basil, geraniums, grasses and other herbs and flowering plants grown throughout the world.
It has many anti-inflammatory properties that help to reduce swelling with insect bites and acts as an insect repellent.

The health benefits within citronella as an essential oil can be accredited to:

❖ Antibacterial elements and may be used as an antibacterial and antiseptic
❖ Its benefits as an antidepressant
❖ Is an antifungal which resists bacterial growth
❖ Will assist with reducing headaches, migraines, tension and depression
❖ May assist with urinary tract infections
❖ Stimulates blood circulation while increasing and stimulating the nervous system
❖ Will assist with prostate and kidney disorders.

As with any medicines, medical advice should always be sought prior to taking or using essential oils.

LEMON GRASS

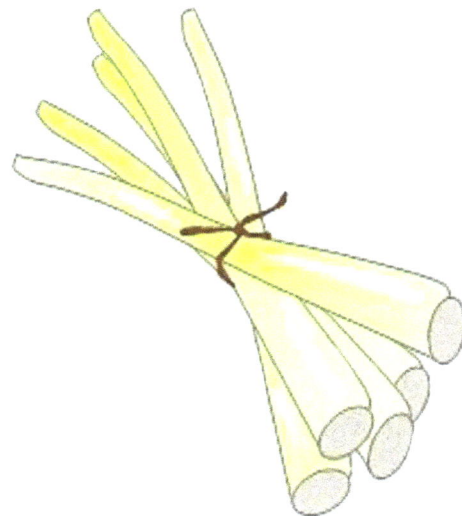

Lemon grass essential oil contains many qualities, most go unnoticed as this oil is normally associated with Thai cooking or Thai related foods.

This remarkable essential oil is used in aromatherapy to:

- ❖ Reduce muscle pain
- ❖ Reduce bodily, including joint, aches and pains
- ❖ To assist with the digestive system and aid stomach discomfort
- ❖ Lemon grass can act as a skin cleanser reducing blotches and lightening the skin
- ❖ It is both an analgesic and antiseptic
- ❖ Has calming properties when applied to the skin through massage or gently rubbing
- ❖ Will reduce nervous tension
- ❖ Assist with sleep disorders
- ❖ Is a natural antidepressant, will support the mind and bring about calming of the human nervous system
- ❖ Through its calming effects, lemon grass has the ability to reduce anxiety; assist to rebuild self-esteem and add to overall wellbeing.

Lemon grass has other benefits: sipped as a tea is refreshing and soothing when added to cake or desert mixes.

A few splashes of lemon grass in a warm bath can work wonders for aching bodies after a hard day of physical work.

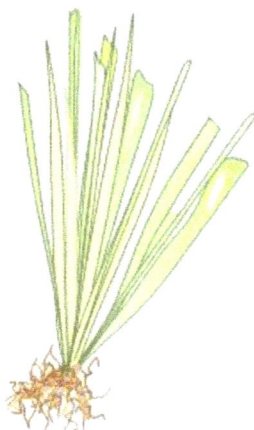

VETIVER

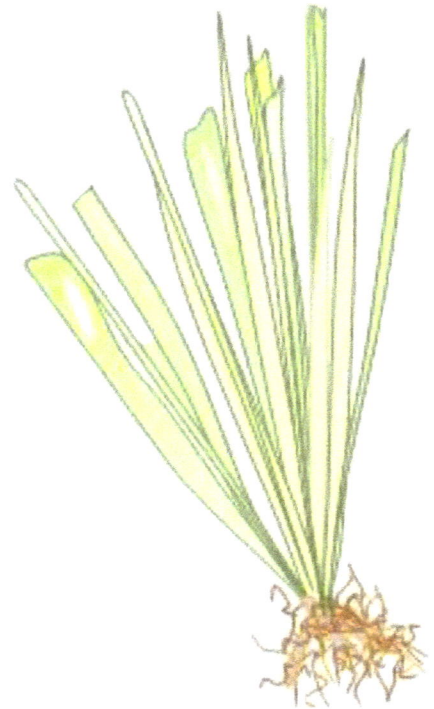

Vetiver is a tropical Indian grass which is cultivated in many countries in Asia. It's known for its fragrant roots which are woven into mats, baskets and fans.

The root is a sweet-scented rhizome, once distilled the rhizome is used in the manufacture of essential oil and perfume.

Vetiver has a calming effect when rubbed into the feet before bedtime. It can also be used to:

- ❖ Strengthen the immune system
- ❖ Calms emotional disturbance
- ❖ Lessens the effects of stress and anxiety
- ❖ If added to a warm bath will reduce muscle tension
- ❖ Is ideal to create grounding when heightened negative feelings are being managed
- ❖ Will assist with erectile dysfunction and stimulate the libido

- ❖ Can be used in hot drinks (check instructions before use).

Vetiver has a rich composite of aromas and is an ideal essential oil when used in aromatherapy. The oil works its wonders when mixed with lavender oil as a massage therapy.

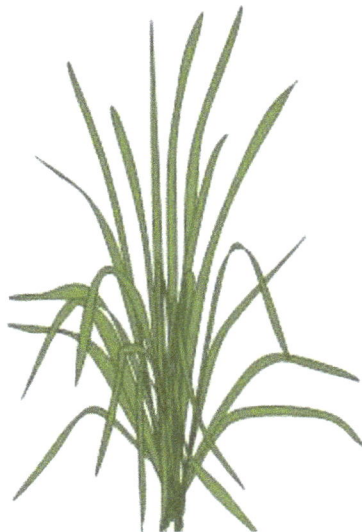

Wood Oils ~ Healing & Wellbeing from Essential Oils

Wood Oils and Their Healing Power

> **Essential Oils**
>
> **Important Essential Oils**
>
> **Wood Oils**
>
> CADE
> CAMPHOR
> CEDARWOOD
> EUCALYPTUS
> SANDALWOOD
> SASSAFRAS
> PINE NEEDLES
> CINNAMON

CADE

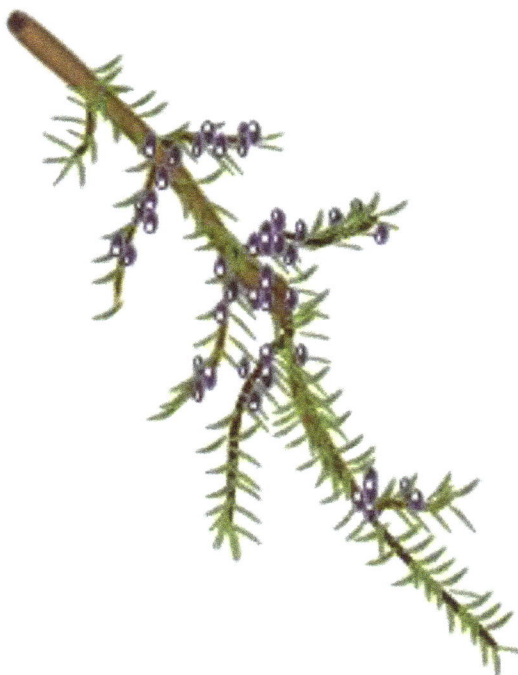

The common name for cade is juniper. The juniper species grows throughout the Northern Hemisphere, the mountains of the tropics and as far down as the equator.

Essential cade oil is distilled from the young twigs and the new wood of the tree. The virgin oil has a distinct tar-like smell. Cade oil was introduced to the French in the 19th Century to treat skin irritation and used as an antiseptic.

The essential oil has benefits to cure:

- ❖ Dermatitis
- ❖ Eczema
- ❖ Psoriasis
- ❖ Hair loss through scalp infections
- ❖ Dandruff and herpes.

Cade oil may be used on animals to help heal:

- ❖ Ulcers
- ❖ Scabies
- ❖ Worms and parasites.

(Seek professional advice before applying it to animals.)

Cade essential oil has been used in prayer, meditation and to balance breathing for thousands of years. The essence from the oil will:

- ✓ Help to heal your mind and memory from pain and hurtful experiences
- ✓ It will help to reduce cravings for drugs, nicotine, and other destructive habits
- ✓ It will help with spiritual support and allow ease and bonding to the higher self and divine universal energies.

Cade oil should be used in low doses and is an effective oil to blend with other oils such as: cinnamon, lemon, rose, geranium and orange.

CAMPHOR

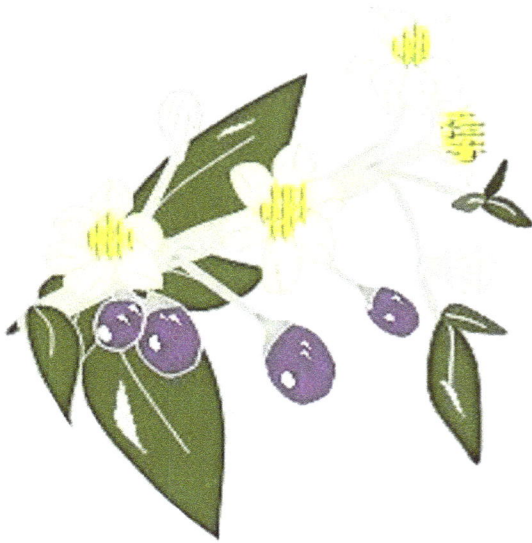

In times of headache or head pain, camphor essential oil contains a natural cooling agent. Apply a mix of camphor and coconut oil to the forehead and back of the neck to relieve pain. Camphor comes from two main trees: the common camphor tree and the Borneo camphor tree.

The main benefits of camphor oil:

- ❖ Prevents skin infections and sores
- ❖ Improves circulation
- ❖ Aids in correcting the metabolism, digestion, and secretion glands of the body
- ❖ Lessons agitation and nervous disorders
- ❖ Eliminates gas or prevents gas forming in the large intestine. If gas forms camphor will help to eliminate it through gentle rubbing of the area
- ❖ Relieves muscle spasms and cramps
- ❖ Increases libido when rubbed externally on the body
- ❖ May help to cure erectile problems; is a powerful stimulant

- ❖ Reduces arthritic pain
- ❖ Relaxes the bodily nervous system, in turn, relaxing the functions of the body and brain
- ❖ Relieves neuralgia
- ❖ Reduces bodily swelling from injury
- ❖ Relieves congestion and bronchial conditions
- ❖ Is effective in supporting the treatment of epilepsy, viral diseases of the reproductive organs.

Other benefits include:

- ✓ When worn in a face mask prevents flu viruses
- ✓ Helps to prevent the measles virus from spreading.

Warning: camphor oil may become addictive if it's overused.

CEDARWOOD

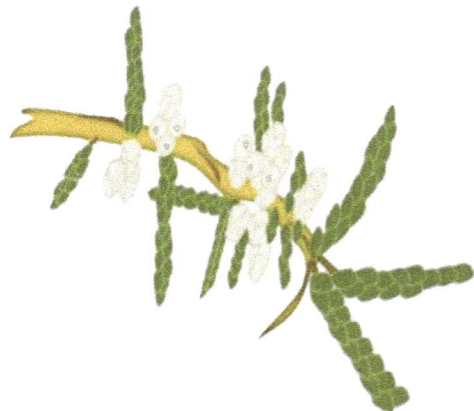

Cedarwood oil has been used since ancient times. It was used by the Egyptians, Tibetans, used throughout Northern American by native Indians and has many mentions in the Bible.

Amongst its many benefits, cedarwood essential oil can improve skin, add lustre and restore hair. Its other properties can:

- ❖ Benefit relaxation
- ❖ Calm nervous tension
- ❖ Promote longevity
- ❖ Relieves bronchial congestion
- ❖ Can cleanse wounds on open skin and ward off infections. To use: mix with antiseptic cream. Do not apply cedar wood essential oil in its natural state
- ❖ Can kill fungal infections
- ❖ Cedarwood essential oil, when mixed with coconut cream, can help to relieve arthritis
- ❖ Inhalation – drop a few drops into hot water when inhaling – this will relieve head colds and ease respiratory infections
- ❖ Will assist in sleep deprivation
- ❖ When rubbed onto the body will tighten and add tone to muscles
- ❖ Improve metabolism.

Cedarwood oil is obtained by distillation of the wood species: *Juniper virginiana.*

A study performed by Dr. Terry Friedmann M.D. and Dennis Eggett from Brigham Young University found that using cedarwood oil on children could greatly improve their focus and learning capacity. Thirty-four children with **ADHD** *were given one of three essential oils (cedarwood, vetiver or lavender) to inhale or nothing at all.*

Children held up a bottle of essential oil to their nostrils and took three deep inhalations three times a day for thirty days. At the end of the study, there were 30 subjects who retook an EEG and T.O.V.A. test. The researchers found that both the vetiver and cedarwood oil groups experienced improvements in brain

activity and reduced the ADHD symptoms.[1]

Use cedarwood oil with caution. Expectant mothers should seek medical advice before using this oil.

EUCALYPTUS

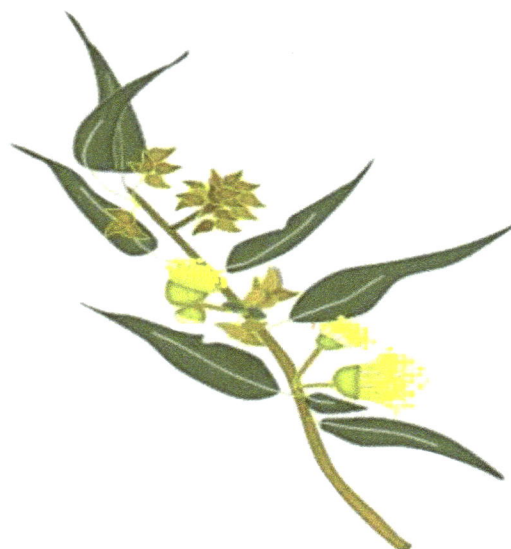

Eucalyptus oil is mainly derived from *E. dives* and *E.globulus.* Both oils are beneficial to healing and wellbeing.

Eucalyptus oil is made from partially dried twigs and young leaves. The oil is extracted through steam distillation.

Eucalyptus oil is beneficial in the treatment of many illnesses including:

- ❖ Sinusitis and bronchial conditions
- ❖ Common cold and flu, including flu like symptoms
- ❖ Pneumonia and its associated conditions including coughs and respiratory infections
- ❖ Asthma and associated conditions
- ❖ Will stimulate the immune system

---

[1] Terry S Friedmann, MD., ABHM

- ❖ Provide antioxidants to the bodily system
- ❖ Is calming to the nervous system
- ❖ Eucalyptus dives[2] can encourage pain relief in trauma
- ❖ Helps to relieve headaches or tension headaches
- ❖ Fights infections
- ❖ Can be used with steam inhalation.

Eucalyptus oil has many benefits when used as an antiviral with conditions including: herpes simplex and other transmitted viruses.

Always seek medical or professional advice before using essential oils as cure for a defined medical condition

SANDALWOOD

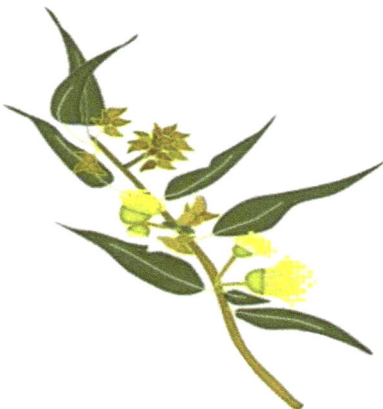

Sandalwood oil is used in essential oils, perfumery and medicines. It's oil is extracted from *Santalum album.* This fragrant wood is considered to be the best of the sandalwood varieties.

The essential oil of sandalwood is extracted through steam distillation. The older the tree, the better the aroma and the oil reserve within the tree.

For centuries, sandalwood has been revered amongst many civilisations and used through both rituals and religious offerings.

As with all other essential oils, it should not be used in its pure form. It can be mixed with fractionated coconut oil to reduce sensitivity to the skin. Sandalwood offers many health benefits which include:

- ❖ Used as an astringent in mouth wash it helps to heal gums and ulcers

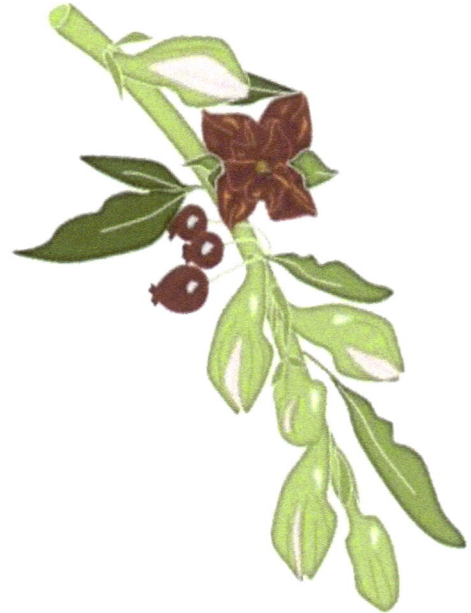

---

[2] Broad-leafed or Blue Peppermint eucalyptus

- ❖ Is an antiseptic for cuts to the skin
- ❖ Helps to heal boils, acne, sores, and pimples
- ❖ Supports the bodily system as an anti-inflammatory. When tension is high, rub the back of the neck and forehead with this essential oil, it helps to sooth the brain and the nervous system. Before use, mix with a carrier oil
- ❖ Helps with the circulatory and excretory systems of the human body
- ❖ Helps with reducing fever from illness, the flu and other fever conditions
- ❖ Sooths insect bites or wounds
- ❖ Helps as a relaxant on muscles and stops muscle spasm and cramps
- ❖ Sandalwood helps to boost memory, keeps the brain cool in times of stress and assists with soothing the nervous system.

Sandalwood has extensive worth as an essential oil. Not only is it calming to the skin, but it can be used as a skin care treatment.

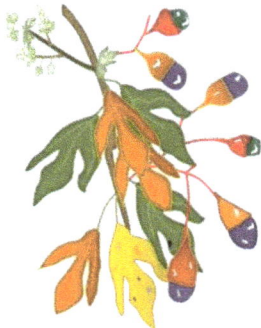

SASSAFRAS

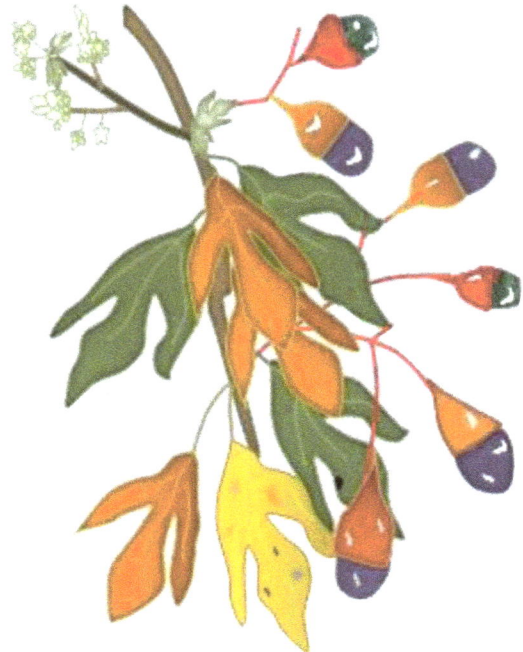

Sassafras oil in its purest form needs to be respected. This oil, when unrefined, can be lethal because it contains safrole. Safrole is a phenylpropene[3] and is banned in many countries. This is a natural product of the plant and protects it from insect invasion.

On the positive side, when used in moderation and with respect, the essential can give many benefits, these include:

- ❖ It helps to reduce painful arthritic problems
- ❖ Helps to reduce blood pressure
- ❖ Will strengthen the immune system, (do not ingest)
- ❖ Will help to reduce headaches and general aches and pains associated with the flu
- ❖ Will assist with pain control with rheumatism and gout

---

[3] Phenylpropene is used in illicit drug manufacturing

- ❖ Has benefits which will boost the immune system which may eliminate the free radicals
- ❖ Will reduce inflammation when rubbed onto the skin externally
- ❖ Can assist with dental care.

Over many centuries sassafras has been used to flavour foods and beverages. Because of its unique flavour and In times gone, sassafras twigs were used as toothbrushes.

Sassafras is a genus of aromatic deciduous trees. Essential oil is extracted from the wood and bark of the American *S. albidum.*

PINE NEEDLES

The oil will support the human system:

- ❖ Steam inhalation to relieve cold and flu symptoms
- ❖ Helps to soothe aching and tired muscles including joints
- ❖ Will improve circulation
- ❖ Can be used on minor cuts and abrasions
- ❖ Will help to clear mucus and increase breathing
- ❖ Helps to improve mental cognition and learning capacity
- ❖ Is an antioxidant
- ❖ Is an anti-inflammatory
- ❖ May support the healing of eczema and psoriasis
- ❖ Will help to heal and stimulate the human system.

Mix a diluted solution of pine needle essential oil with a carrier oil and rub onto the areas of the body after sport, distance walking, or strenuous exercise, this is both beneficial to the mind and body.

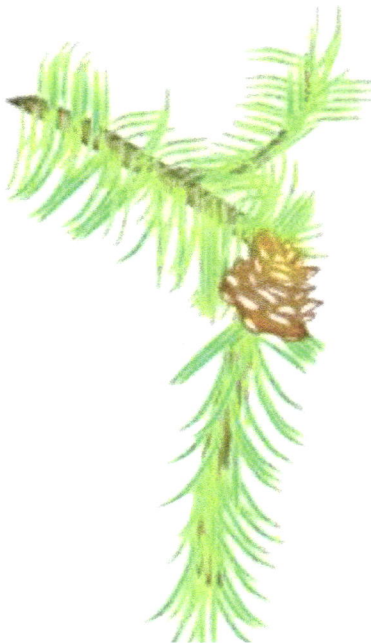

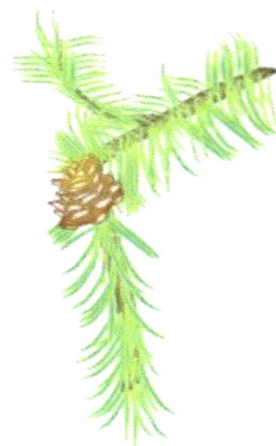

Pine needle essential oil is extracted from the *Pinus sylvestris* pine tree and is steam distilled. Essential oils are made from the needles, twigs, and cones. Pine has many qualities including relieving mental fatigue and nervous tension. This oil should be used in moderation and not used on sensitive skin.

CINNAMON

Cinnamon essential oil is extracted from the bark of the cinnamon tree *Laurus cinnamomum*. Cinnamon oil, when inhaled tends to be warming, energizing and is stimulating to our senses. Cinnamon oil offers some respite to the many maladies that we experience throughout our daily lives. The benefits of this oil include:

- ❖ When stomach or gut disorders cause discomfort, gently rub the area with a few drops of cinnamon and coconut oil to bring relief
- ❖ It helps to boost emotions and works well as an anti-depressant
- ❖ It fights many infections, including foot infections such as athletes' foot
- ❖ Is an effective treatment against head lice
- ❖ Helps to prevent nausea and indigestion
- ❖ Helps to prevent catching the flu and the common cold
- ❖ Cinnamon essential oil helps to stimulate the libido and arouse sexual interest
- ❖ Fights bad cholesterol allowing comfort to return. (Seek medical advice before self-medicating)
- ❖ Fights many infections and bacteria
- ❖ Stimulates the immune system

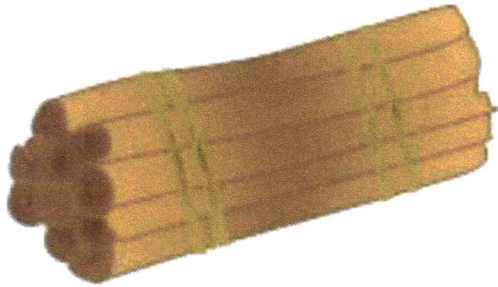

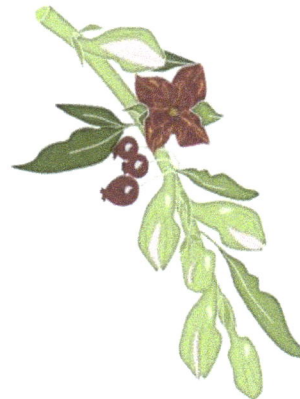

- ❖ Has a high antioxidant content.

There are many benefits offered by this essential oil. With head lice, take care when using it on children. Use a breakdown of 4 drops of cinnamon oil, 10 drops of vinegar and 10 drops of water make a solution; use when rinsing the hair.

It's time to take a break.....

Breathing ~ The Joy
Further Techniques to Manage Stressful Times

As Before:

1. Make sure your jaw is relaxed – unclench your jaw right now and feel the difference
2. Your feet and legs are uncrossed
3. Your shoulders are loose and not tense.

- ✓ Breathe in through your nose – hold: count to 3
- ✓ Push the air down into your lungs – hold: count to 3
- ✓ Exhale the stale air through your mouth – hold: count of three – then start the process again.

To Increase Your Wellbeing:

- ❖ Do the above breathing exercises: breathe in through your nose and count to 3 and then exhale allowing 3 counts. As you do this exercise regularly, you will develop a rhythm that will allow you to focus more deeply on the breathing journey you are on.
- ❖ Now take your breathing journey (with the 3 counts) to 20 times: breathing in 3 – breathing out 3.
- ❖ Concentrate on doing this exercise 20 times. Once this is done you are ready to go to the next level. Maintain the breathing rhythm
- ❖ NOW
- ❖ Concentrate on your breathing and count down from 50, 49, 48 until you reach 1.

Breathing ~ The Joy

Further Techniques to Manage Stressful Times Cont.,

When you have finished your breathing exercises, you would have completed 70 revitalising and energising gifts you have given yourself. Your exercises are just for you. It's sometimes difficult to find the time to complete these gifts so I do mine when I get into bed at night.

This process of meditation is good for my heart, mind and soul.

By using your favourite essential oil at the time of doing the breathing exercises adds to a great comfort that is mine and mine alone.

Remember, you can do breathing exercises at any time: day or night…

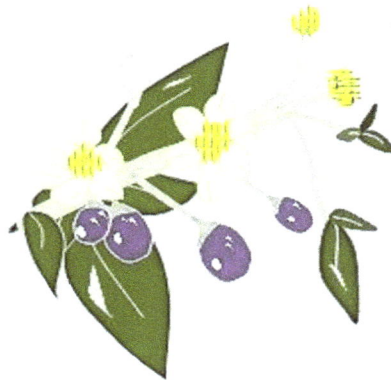

A Poem ~

Eucalyptus

Eucalyptus trees are these with their wood,
bark, and leaves...

For their perfume and scent hangs there as it
lingers within the fresh breeze and the cool
autumn air...

These precious plants have healing oil ~
you walk through the bush, you stop ~ you may
sneeze...!

Their perfume or scent can be strong ~ but that
is all part of the bushland song...

Millions of years have passed for these magical
gifts to evolve...

It is now our good blessing that many health
problems will they solve...!

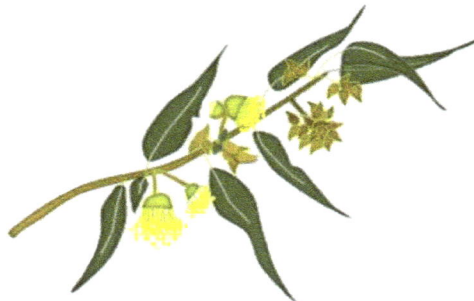

Flavouring Oils
~
Healing &
Wellbeing from
Essential
Oils

Flavouring Oils and Their Healing Power

Essential Oils

Important Essential Oils

Flavouring Oils

PEPPERMINT
SPEARMINT
STAR ANISE
CELERY
CLOVES
LEMON
ORANGE
LIME
CARAWAY
NUTMEG
THYME

The following essential oils, though used as flavourings, are used to aid and assist healing in the human body.

PEPPERMINT

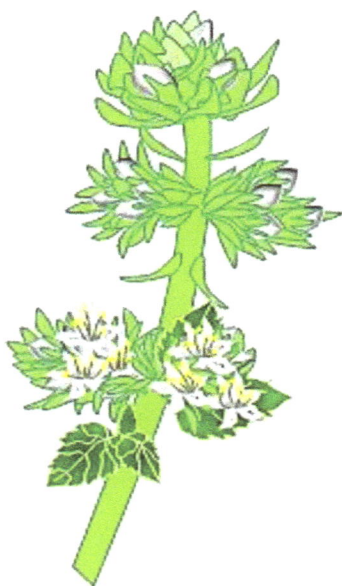

Peppermint oil is a hybrid species resulting from a combination of spearmint and water mint (*Mentha aquatic*). Accordingly, the oil has been found in Egyptian pyramids dating back as far as 1,000 BC. The oil is also reputedly used in ancient Japanese and Chinese folk medicine. The peppermint plant sits in both the flavouring and herb camps when classified as an essential oil.

The benefits of peppermint oil are many, some uses include:

- ❖ Relieves muscle and joint pain (apply oil externally to painful areas)
- ❖ Will help to relax muscles and muscular tension when made into a tea
- ❖ Helps to relieve stomach cramps due to period pain
- ❖ Will assist with relieving IBS pain
- ❖ When inhaled as a steam inhalation, helps to relieve colds and flu symptoms
- ❖ Helps to sooth respiratory infections
- ❖ When used in a vaporiser, helps to reduce tension headaches and sinusitis or Rub two drops on a tissue and rub on the temple and back of the neck
- ❖ Will give seasonal allergy relief
- ❖ Will increase energy and maximise energy performance in sport when inhaled prior to the event
- ❖ Has antiseptic properties and helps to reduce swelling
- ❖ Has proven benefits in helping to improve circulation
- ❖ Helps to improve overall skin health
- ❖ Will improve colic symptoms in young children
- ❖ Helps to reduce halitosis and other breath conditions.

If persistent unpleasant odour comes from the mouth, seek medical or clinical advice.

Essential peppermint oil has many natural benefits. Like many of the oils mentioned, always seek medical or professional advice before using them.

SPEARMINT

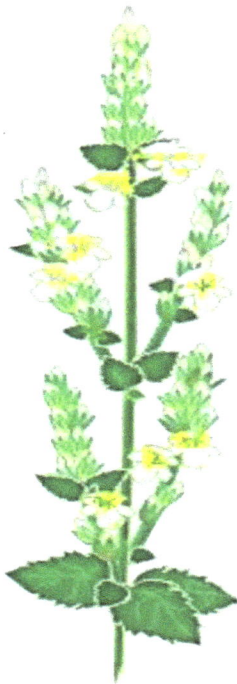

Spearmint essential oil is gentle oil when compared to peppermint oil. Spearmint has only 0.5% of menthol whereas peppermint carries a 40% of menthol composition. Children and elderly folk find spearmint softer and kinder to their skin and more palatable on the tongue.

Spearmint, among other mints, grows around the Mediterranean and was thought to be brought to Britain by the Romans.
Spearmint is primarily known for its flavour enhancement in food and beverages. The aromatic essences are refreshing and uplifting.
The beneficial uses of this essential oil are many including:

❖ Help to remedy constipation and irregular bowel movements including the expulsion of unwanted gases
❖ Assists with easing asthma and breathing difficulties
❖ Will assist with reducing sinusitis and respiratory ailments
❖ Will help to reduce the symptoms of the common cold and bronchitis
❖ Assists with alleviating Indigestion
❖ Skin problems, will soothe irritation (only use with an oil carrier such as coconut oil)
❖ May assist with dental problems, including tooth ache
❖ Helps to remedy headaches and migraines
❖ May assist with depression and mood swings
❖ Will help with mental focus especially under stressful conditions for teenagers when taking examinations
❖ When used in aromatherapy, will assist with relieving stress, muscle tension and fatigue
❖ Antifungal properties for feet problems
❖ Restorative properties assisting in body and nerve repair
❖ Is an immune boosting oil adding to overall wellbeing.

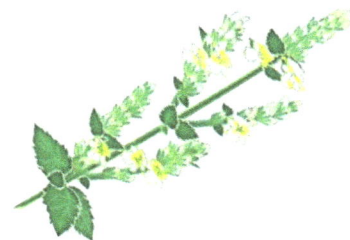

STAR ANISE

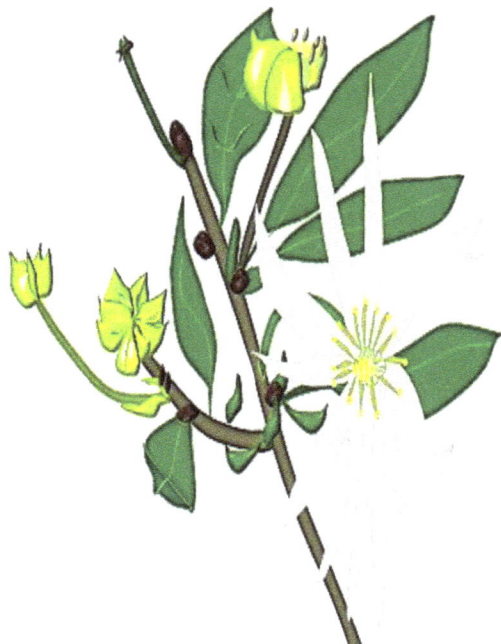

Anise oil may have a narcotic effect and should be used with caution. Use this essential oil as a calming oil when feeling stressed or if anxiety is taking a grip.

Other benefits of this little star include:

- ❖ It can assist to diminish headaches and neuralgia pain
- ❖ Will assist with digestion or gas flatulence
- ❖ Is calming and may be used as a sedative before bedtime. Mix with a carrier oil, dab a little oil on a tissue and rub over the forehead and back of the neck
- ❖ Used in the morning, it may act as a stimulant and assist in clearing the head
- ❖ Will slow down the circulation through its calming and sedative effects in anxious or stressful environments
- ❖ May assist with hypertension

- ❖ May treat respiratory disorders and assist with breathing difficulties.

Anise has many benefits, if you feel the flu coming on use star anise to help fight the virus. If feeling life pressures, keep a bottle handy to lift your spirits. Dab a little on a tissue and use when needed. Like all essential oils use in moderation.

CELERY

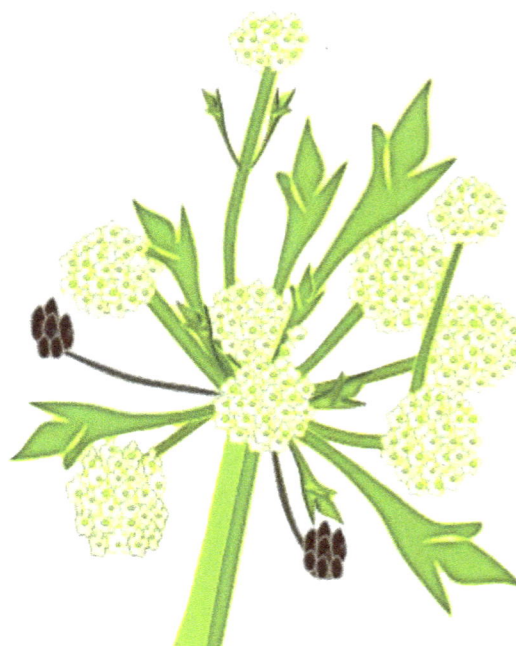

The plant is related to the wild carrot family. The oil used in essential oils is extracted from the celery flower when it seeds. Celery seed oil has many uses including its use in aromatherapy and relief in arthritic conditions. Other benefits include:

- ❖ Relief from rheumatism
- ❖ Relief from gout and joint stiffness
- ❖ Amenorrhea (an absence in menstruation for at least six months in a woman who previously had normal periods) The essential oil may help periods to normalise, if in doubt, seek medical attention

- ❖ Relief of indigestion
- ❖ Relief with sciatica.

Celery seed oil can help to detoxify the human system. It can help to stimulate the kidneys to eradicate toxins that contribute to the build-up of kidney stones.

By mixing the celery oil with a carrier oil, such as coconut oil, the mixture can be rubbed into the lower abdominal area aiding detoxification. A few drops added to a warm bath can also assist with relaxation assisting with in lowering blood pressure and hypertension.

CLOVES

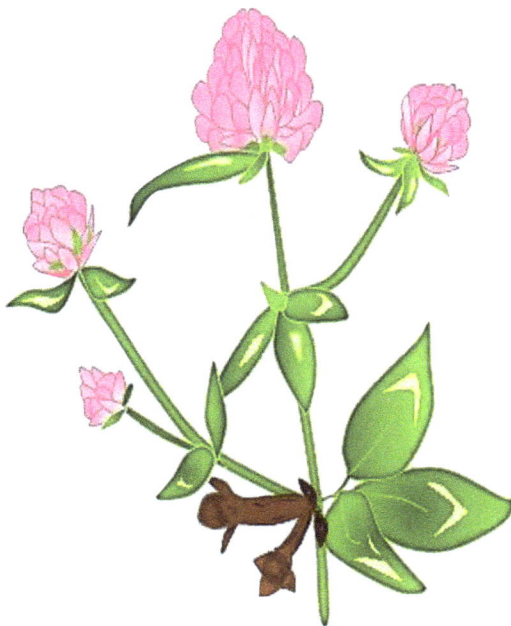

Clove oil is extracted from the dried flower buds of *Eugenia Caryophyllata*. The oil contains many benefits for the human body these include:

- ❖ Is an anaesthetic and used in toothache
- ❖ Has both an antimicrobial and antifungal properties and other stimulating benefits for the human system

- ❖ May be used as an aphrodisiac
- ❖ It can assist to heal skin issues or pimple breakouts
- ❖ It has antiviral properties and assists with the prevention of colds and flu
- ❖ Will help to ease coughs and asthma
- ❖ May be used to ease indigestion
- ❖ When used in bathing, clove oil will assist with easing stress and the related muscle tension caused by stress.

Cloves are thought to have been one of the first spices traded over 1,500 BC. The use of cloves is found in both Roman and Chinese ancient writings.

LEMONS

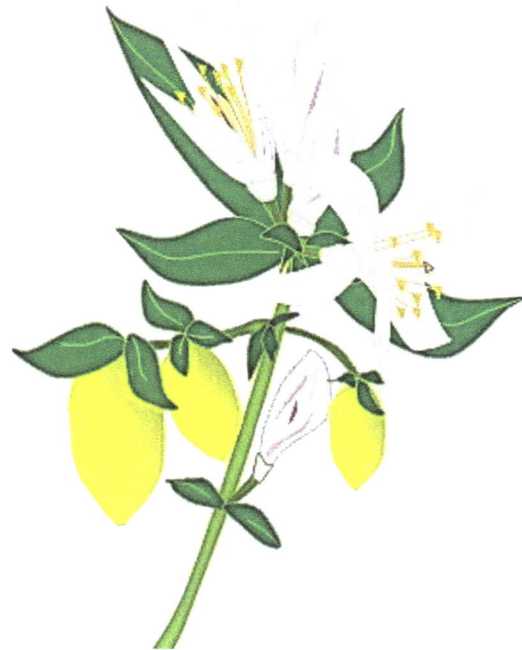

Lemons are a diverse and versatile fruit; with so much to offer for wellbeing and general health. Not only are they good for healthy hair, nails, and skin but they are so very good for cleaning the blood.

In order to stay healthy, the blood alkaline/acid balance needs to be maintained – by removing toxins, a lemon drink can help to re-balance blood chemistry and keep blood clean.

Lemons and their oil have been used widely for more than a thousand years. Lemon essential oil is extracted from the cold-pressed lemon peel and not from the fruit.

Essential lemon oil has the ability to increase concentration, therefore allowing creative energy and inspiration to flow.

Other benefits of lemon essential oil include:

* It has powerful antioxidant properties allowing the complete body, brain and mind to be refreshed
* In times of sickness, it will help to drain lymphatic glands
* Has the ability to increase energy
* Will help to fight bacteria in skin breakouts
* Has the ability to reduce fungi and odour with foot conditions
* Relieves coughs and colds
* Will assist with nausea and vomiting during pregnancy (lemon inhalation during times of sickness has proven effective when the feeling of vomiting and nausea are prominent)
* Will help to reduce stress and anxiety during times of stress. Defuse with an atomiser and spray the body prior to busy and stressful days
* For constipation and other gut problems, gently massage the lower back and stomach with lemon essential oil to gain relief

* Nourish the skin by using a dab of lemon essential oil mixed with rosemary before applying makeup.

Lemon essential oil has many advantages for the human bodily system; not only will its scent make your mouth water but it has effective antibacterial and antifungal properties to help keep the human system free from the damage of chemicals, viruses and harm.

ORANGES

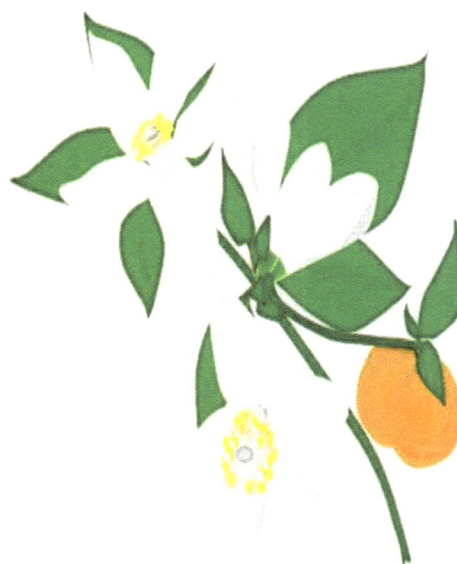

Oranges have many qualities: they are a delicious fruit to eat; they release a lovely bouquet when their skin is broken, and they produce a fine essential oil. Like the lemon, the essential oil is extracted from the peel of the fruit. The sweet orange used in the extraction of essential oil is *Citrus sinensis.*

The use of orange essential oil goes back over thousands of years. The people of China, India, Middle East and the Mediterranean know the benefits of this time-tested oil.

Oranges and orange essential oil are excellent to help ease:

- ❖ The common cold and coughs
- ❖ Is an anti-inflammatory
- ❖ Is a diuretic and helps to keep the urinary tract clean
- ❖ Is a sedative and will help to rectify sleep dis-orders
- ❖ It works as an antiseptic
- ❖ Has calming qualities
- ❖ It will improve skin disorders and promote clearer skin
- ❖ Is effective in aiding and reducing depression
- ❖ Will assist with digestive disorders
- ❖ Will assist with cognitive sharpness and improve attention span
- ❖ The monoterpene compound within oranges has proposed anti-tumour and anti-cancer benefits
- ❖ Oranges and orange essential oil have immune boosting properties.

The treasure trove of health benefits produced by this one fruit is too great to be overlooked.

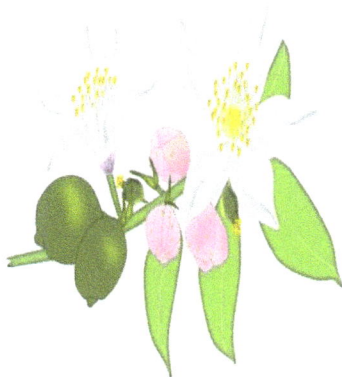

LIMES

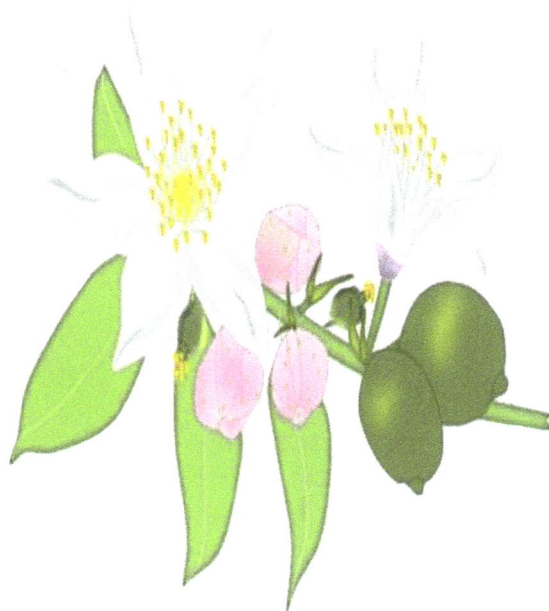

Limes have, within this green treasure trove, a multitude of benefits for the human body. Just by looking at a lime, you can feel the salivation in your mouth start to work.

Essential lime oil is extracted by cold compression or by distillation of its dried peel.

Limes like lemons are full of antioxidants and like many of the citrus fruits fights viral infections.

Limes are beneficial to the human system in many ways, these include:

- ❖ Helps to fight fatigue
- ❖ Stimulates cognition allowing thinking to be clearer allowing clarity to take place
- ❖ Helps to reduce anxiety and refreshes the tired mind after exhaustive mind work as in sitting for examinations
- ❖ Will assist with clearing skin and skin breakouts – teenagers may benefit with a

dab of geranium and lime oil blended with coconut oil onto troublesome acne

- ❖ Is an anti-viral
- ❖ Will help to reduce fever and flu-like symptoms
- ❖ Will assist with curing bronchitis
- ❖ Is an antiseptic
- ❖ Will assist with detoxification of the human system
- ❖ Aids digestion of food
- ❖ May assist with colon disorders
- ❖ Will help to clean and refresh the urinary tract reducing urinary tract infections
- ❖ Helps to prevent bacterial infections
- ❖ Assists with blood coagulation.

A blend of lime, rose, and orange with coconut oil assists in fighting aging when applied to the skin.
This oil blends well with bergamot, cedarwood and grapefruit.

As an essential oil used in aromatherapy, like many oils mentioned in this book, it will relax tight muscles, help with clearing congestion, and allow the mind to find peace.

The treasure trove of the lime is used in many foods and beverages.

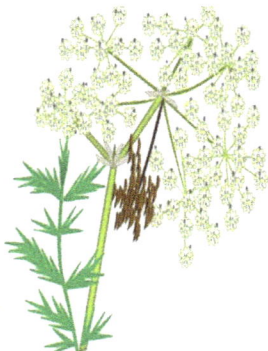

CARAWAY

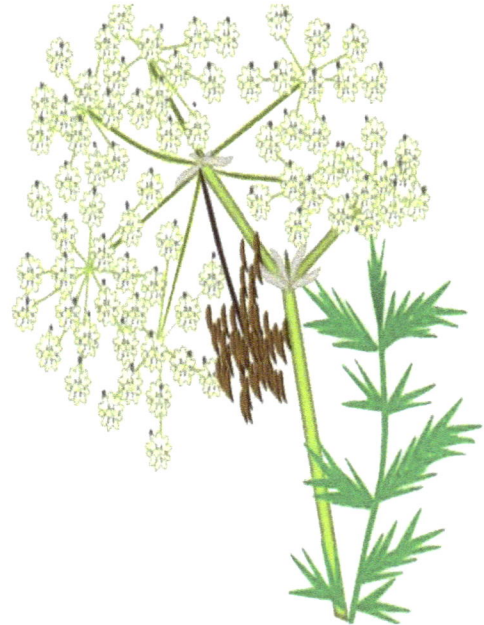

Caraway seeds and essential oils have many benefits for the human body, brain, and mind.

Essential caraway oil is extracted from the tiny seed of the plant. Caraway essential oil when used in aromatherapy helps to calm the nervous system, relieve stress and calm the mind. Other uses include:

- ❖ Can be used as an antihistamine
- ❖ Will support the human system by alleviating spasmodic episodes in coughing bouts
- ❖ Helps to prevent bacteria and microbes from infecting the skin
- ❖ Helps to relieve menstruation and menopausal discomfort
- ❖ Caraway oil will relieve gas, gut discomfort in children and adults. Rub a little oil onto the stomach and gentle rub in a circular motion.

Other uses of caraway oil and seeds:

- ❖ Caraway oil diluted in milk or a warm drink supports the heart and cardiac health; it helps to maintain heart strength, strengthens heart muscles, and helps to prevent hardening of the arteries
- ❖ The oil helps to reduce blood pressure and lowers cholesterol
- ❖ For mothers' breast feeding: caraway oil and seeds are known to increase milk production. During this period of breast feeding it keeps the infant safe from flatulence and indigestion.

Caraway oil is an antiseptic and has disinfectant properties.

NUTMEG

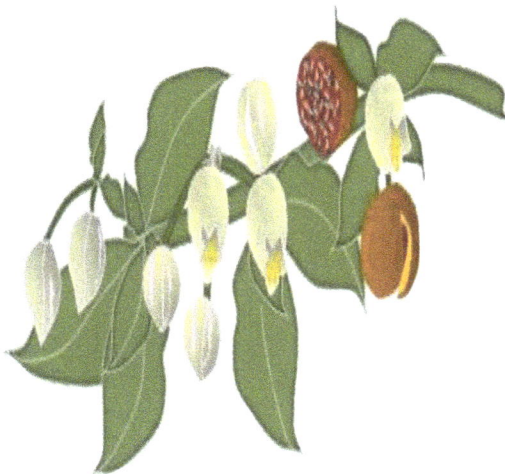

Nutmeg essential oil like all other oils should be used in moderation. This oil has been used over centuries as a spice it does however have other great benefits. Nutmeg is known to stimulate the nervous system thus enhancing your brain's performance capacity. It adds to enhancing concentration and contributes to memory skill building.
Nutmeg essential oil will help in work performance and output, assist with examination performance, and contribute to brain and mind health.

Other benefits of nutmeg include:

- ❖ Treating cardiovascular disease
- ❖ Viral and bacterial infections
- ❖ Urinary tract inflammation
- ❖ Digestive disorders
- ❖ Impotency in males
- ❖ Joint and muscular pain
- ❖ Hormonal imbalance
- ❖ Menstrual cramps and such painful effects including backache caused by period pain
- ❖ Respiratory conditions, including asthma
- ❖ Low blood pressure
- ❖ Helps to reduce insomnia.

Indian and Chinese cultures have known of the therapeutic properties of this ancient spice. It's now a valued oil and is used widely in aromatherapy.

When used in massage, nutmeg essential oil helps to relieve muscle pain; it promotes circulation to damaged areas of the body and works as a natural painkiller.

THYME

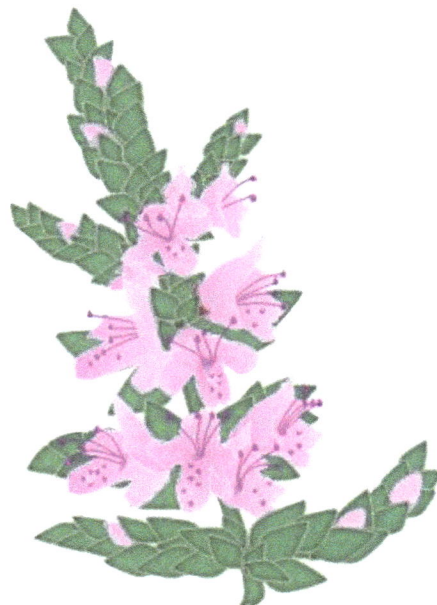

more than a culinary extra when cooking the Sunday roast.

Thyme essential oil is obtained from the leaves of the plant.

The oil is used in aromatherapy. When stress or anxiety is high, use a little thyme to reduce stress and anxiety. Thyme has an active substance called carvacrol; this is thought to support neuron activity within the human system, including the human brain.

Other benefits of thyme essential oil include:

- ❖ Calming for the gut and intestine
- ❖ Can reduce high blood pressure
- ❖ Can be used to help lower cholesterol
- ❖ Is effective when used to rehydrate the skin and helps to reduce acne, pimples, and skin breakouts
- ❖ Will help to reduce diarrhoea
- ❖ Reduce cramps and aches
- ❖ Will support the reduction of pain from arthritis
- ❖ Has benefits in reducing colic
- ❖ Will help to ease a sore throat
- ❖ Will assist with easing coughing and bronchitis
- ❖ Will support the gut by reducing flatulence
- ❖ Can be used as a diuretic to increase urination.

Thyme contains both vitamins A and C; these vitamins help to support the immune system.

With this herb, research is underway into the positive effects of protecting the bowel from colon cancer.

Thyme has been used for thousands of years. The Egyptians used it to embalm their dead and the Romans to protect their food from spoiling. Thyme oil was used by the Romans to counteract poisons if their food was tampered with. If they thought they were suffering from poison, they would bath in a thyme bath.

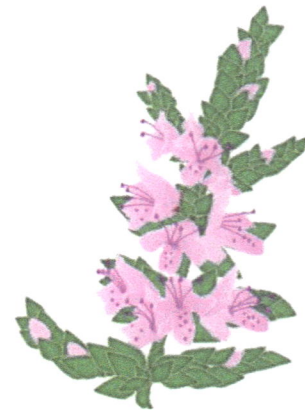

It's time to take a break.....

Marmalade Recipe Using Oranges and a Lemon

EQUIPMENT:

- 1 large saucepan
- 5 300 ml sterilised glass jars with secure lids
- Ladle to deliver the hot liquid to the funnel
- Large opening funnel to fill the jars.

INGREDIENTS:

- 8 oranges
- 1 lemon
- 6 dessert spoons of quality gelatin (when adding gelatin to any recipe, buy pure, unflavoured 225 bloom gelatin). This is a high-grade, uncontaminated, product
- 7 dessert spoons of quality organic honey.

METHOD:

1. Squeeze oranges and lemon to remove all juice
2. Cut all of the peel into finely cut pieces – the size of traditional marmalade pieces, very small
3. Combine the peel and juice in a large saucepan
4. Add the honey and stir, continue to stir
5. Place on the stove and bring to just under boiling – (do not boil) continue to stir
6. Turn the heat down to simmer and simmer for about one hour – (until fruit is soft) – continue to stir
7. Once simmered, allow to cool, no longer than 5 minutes
8. Stir in the gelatin in small, individual spoonful
9. Fill the jars with the slightly cooled mixture
10. Allow to cool for a further 5 minutes
11. Secure lids to jars while warm
12. As this marmalade has no preservatives: keep in refrigerator.

This is a refreshing, healthy treat that can be eaten at any time – day or night. The peel contains many anti-cancer and anti-viral benefits. Worldwide research is ongoing to the benefits of citrus peel.

Poem ~

Oranges & Lemons

Oranges and lemons are humble fruits ~ their healing power we cannot dispute...

They grow in warmer climates around the world and for thousands of years their story has not unfurled ~

It is now time to reveal the power they have to eal ~ The health benefits they give and the way they make us feel ~

Money cannot be compared to the goodness and richness they hold...

For their story of evolution is still to be told...

Such health benefits they offer and healing to show and possibly the reason why they don't grow in the snow...!

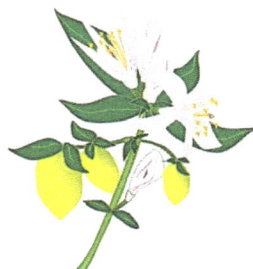

Herb Oils ~ Healing & Wellbeing from Essential Oils

Herb Oils and Their Healing Power

> ## *Essential Oils*
>
> **Important Essential Oils**
>
> **Herb Oils**
>
> BASIL
> CORIANDER
> OREGANO
> ROSEMARY
> PARSLEY
> CHAMOMILE
> HOPS

Like the flavouring oils, herb oils are part of the collection of essential oils used in healing.

BASIL

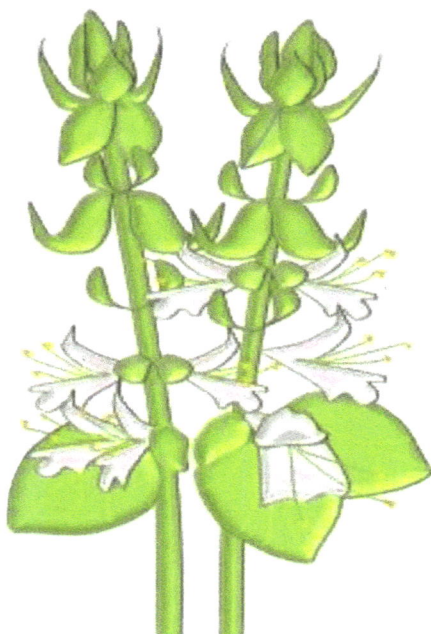

The leaves and seeds of the basil plant are essential to the medicinal value of basil essential oil.

Basil is used as a culinary herb worldwide.

Emotionally and spiritually basil essential oil can be used to ground and bring about peace to the human being through interacting with the nervous system and connecting to the human psyche. Basil essential oil has the power to help to renew, bring about calmness and reduce stress.

Other benefits of this oil include:

- ❖ Applying to sore and tired muscles – this allows the muscle to slowly relax
- ❖ Apply to sore and aching feet; this will help to fight fatigue
- ❖ It will help to prevent nausea and motion sickness
- ❖ Inhaling the essence when added to steam inhalation will help to alleviate congestion, bronchitis, and head colds
- ❖ Has benefits for treating asthma and other respiratory conditions
- ❖ Will improve digestion
- ❖ Can be applied to cuts and wounds (seek medical advice)
- ❖ Will help to rectify skin conditions such as acne
- ❖ Has benefits to help reduce stomach cramps, bloating and loosen the bowel relieving constipation
- ❖ Will help to reduce melancholia and depression
- ❖ Helps to increase blood circulation and increase the metabolism of the human system
- ❖ Promotes alertness during times of stress and fatigue.

Basil essential oil mixes well with clove, bergamot, geranium, lemon, rosemary and lavender.

It contains the vitamins magnesium, iron and calcium.

CORIANDER

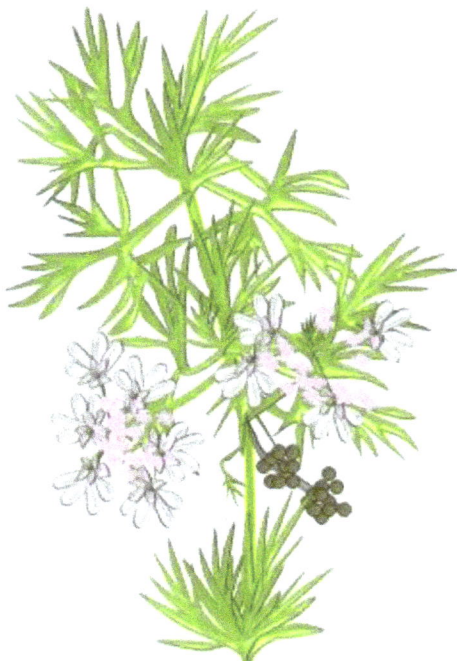

Coriander or cilantro, as it's sometimes called in different parts of the world, relate to the seeds and leaves of the plant.

Coriander oil is extracted from the seed by steam distillation. While coriander is known as a food flavouring herb its health benefits as an essential oil are numerous. These benefits include:

- ❖ Re-establish personal boundaries which may have been broken down through intimidation, harassment or bullying
- ❖ Helps with emotional re-balancing
- ❖ While used in massage, will assist with reducing joint inflammation, muscle stiffness or soreness
- ❖ Will tone and rejuvenate the skin when used after bath or showering
- ❖ Helps with balancing hormones through times of stress
- ❖ Assists the digestive system
- ❖ Acts as a stimulant to create extra physical energy
- ❖ Can assist with reducing mood swings from bad to good moods
- ❖ Will support insulin response
- ❖ Will help to reduce coughing and assist with breathing when experiencing bronchial infections
- ❖ Helps to reduce muscle cramping in times of extreme sport
- ❖ Supports healing and acts as an antifungal when rubbed into sore, rough or broken skin on injured feet
- ❖ Is used as an aphrodisiac.

If you want to boost your married life or relationship, use coriander oil to help you on your journey.

The oil mixes well with bergamot, cinnamon, ginger, and sandalwood.

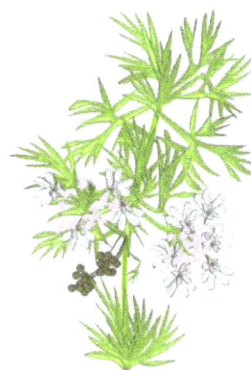

OREGANO

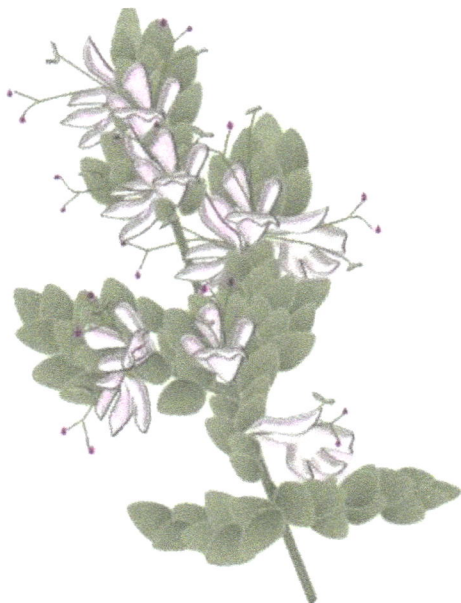

Oregano essential oil has many benefits including the power to assist with concentration.

This sweet-scented oil is extracted from the leaves of the plant by steam distillation.

Accordingly, oregano oil has undergone research which has shown that it has fundamental and greater oxygen absorption capacity than any other fruit or vegetable oil.[4]

Oregano essential oil is known as effective, antimicrobial oil, therefore works as a natural antibiotic. Having said that, always seek professional advice if you have concerns.

This herb was originally used to preserve food, but its wider uses have come down as knowledge through the centuries. Oregano essential oil has

active properties which include its ability to help with:

❖ Lowering cholesterol
❖ May treat yeast or associated infections
❖ Is a powerful antioxidant helping to stop oxidisation of cells (please see footnote, this page)
❖ May assist with improving gut and intestinal health
❖ Can assist with fighting inflammatory infections
❖ May assist with losing weight
❖ Could help to relieve soreness and muscle spasm associated with pain.

This tiny herb offers so many benefits to the human and animal population. Like so many herbs and essential oils mentioned in this book, these tiny flowers and plants need to be revered and appreciated.

ROSEMARY

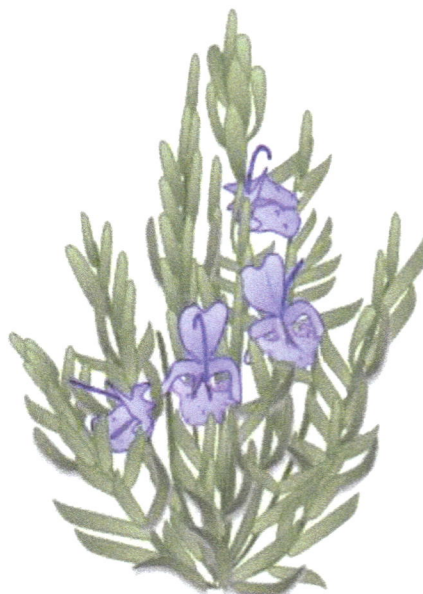

Rosemary essential oil, like so many of the oils, comes with its own

---

[4] : Oxidation is a chemical reaction that can produce free radicals, thereby leading to chain reactions that may damage the cells of organisms.

credentials of benefits. It has been known over many generations that rosemary oil assists with hair re-growth. Another benefit of this oil is the massaging of the scalp to remove dandruff, dead skin and help to heal scalp abrasions.

Other attributes the oil offers are:

- ❖ It stimulates brain and memory capacity allowing greater cognition under times of stress. Is ideal used in a diffuser when tests or examinations are due
- ❖ Overall, helps with memory function
- ❖ Helps to regulate bladder functions
- ❖ Assists with liver detoxification
- ❖ Supports gallbladder function
- ❖ It helps to relieve fatigue and tiredness brought on by heavy workloads
- ❖ Will assist with relaxation when added to a warm bath
- ❖ Will help to reduce the symptoms of coughs and colds
- ❖ Gives relief from headaches when inhaled through steam inhalation or when inhaled from a tissue
- ❖ Works wonders when applied to a gentle foot massage.

Like so many oils, rosemary has its uniqueness and applies itself to the health and wellbeing needs we have.

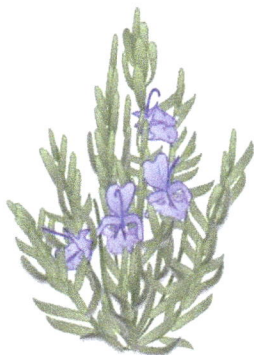

PARSLEY

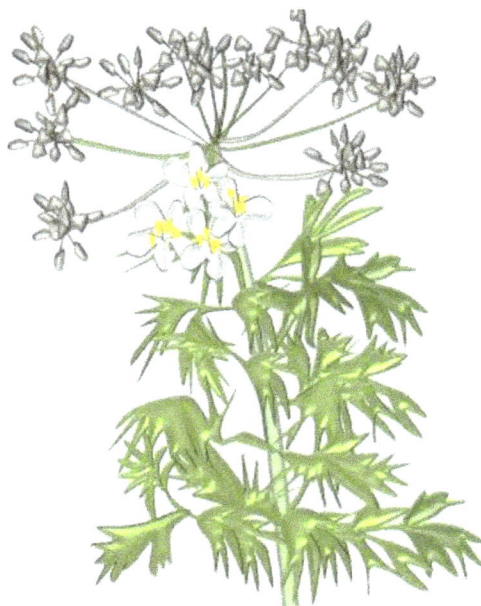

Parsley so commonly associated with culinary delights, and garnishes has great benefits as an essential oil benefiting the human-race with health and wellbeing.

This essential oil has many attributes including its effectiveness on calming the human system when it's under attack from stress and anxiety.

Other benefits of this oil include:

- ❖ Can assist with digestion and give relief to the gut
- ❖ Give relief to arthritic pain and discomfort
- ❖ May assist in cleaning and keeping cuts or abrasions free from infection. Therefore, will lessen the possibility of sepsis
- ❖ When parsley essential oil is applied to the body it will assist the skin and muscle to contract allowing for firmness and a younger appearance
- ❖ Improves flatulence and wind problems in the gut
- ❖ Will help to detoxify the body and clean the blood

- ❖ Will assist with regulating menstruation and relieving cramps
- ❖ Will help to reduce fever and associated conditions
- ❖ Can assist with lowering blood pressure or hypertension
- ❖ May help to relieve constipation
- ❖ Can assist with haemorrhoids
- ❖ Will stimulate libido
- ❖ Is effective in reducing the effects of cystitis.

Parsley essential oil holds clear and significant benefits when used for health and wellbeing. Such a versatile essential oil works with the whole body including the nervous system. The oil works on the circulation of blood throughout the body keeping the human system healthy this helps to keep you energetic, alert and feeling well.

CHAMOMILE

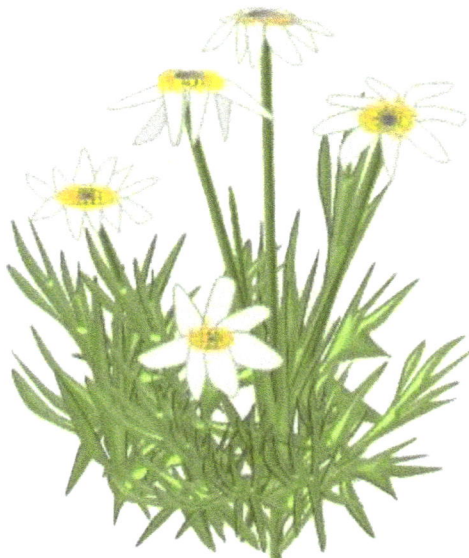

Chamomile essential oil has been used for its calming and soothing qualities over many centuries. In years past, chamomile lotion was applied to stings, insect bites which in turn the lotion relieved the itching.

Chamomile essential oil has many qualities which can contribute to daily health. Not only is chamomile effective in treating insect bites but it works equally well as an anti-depressant.

Other benefits of this ageless oil are:

- ❖ By steam inhalation or dabs on a tissue, chamomile oil is effective in reducing mood swings: from anger to calming
- ❖ Through massage and stimulation Is anti-inflammatory and removes toxins from the human system
- ❖ Assists with relieving depression and sadness. A massage with this oil will help to re-establish self-worth and self-harmony
- ❖ Improves digestion
- ❖ A massage or gently rubbing the inflamed area will assist with rheumatic pain and discomfort
- ❖ When used in aromatherapy, will help to relax tense and tired muscles
- ❖ Will assist with skin care and reduce ageing.
- ❖ Will help to reduce skin blemishes, spot marks and scarring
- ❖ Can assist with removing gas and gut discomfort.

Other benefits from this remarkable oil include it helps as a sedative when used just before bedtime.

HOPS

hair appearance leaving hair shining and healthy
- ❖ May be used as part of a natural remedy in the treatment of psoriasis
- ❖ Will help to relieve tension headaches.

Hop essential oil is a versatile oil that offers many benefits. When using this oil, monitor and measure your reaction to how you feel and respond and how your skin reacts.

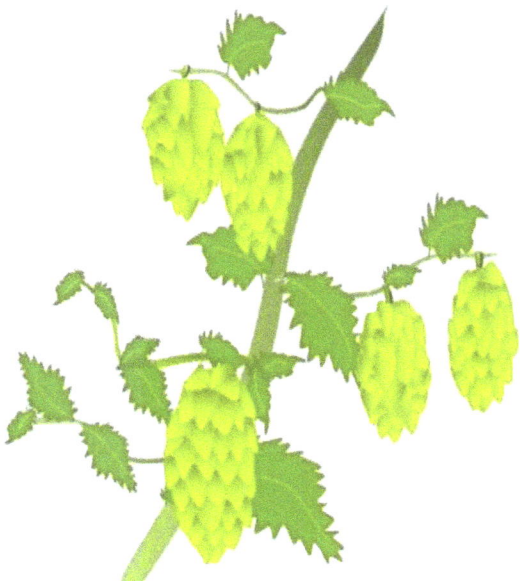

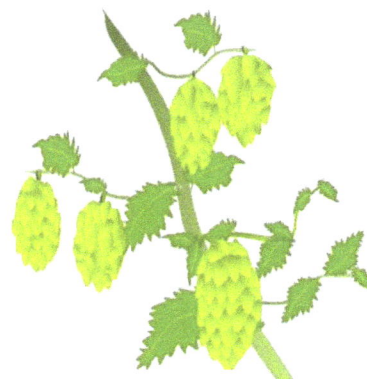

Hops have been used as a medicinal for centuries. Not only are hops renowned for the taste in different beers but they are known for their sedative effects when insomnia is present.

Hop essential oil is effective when used as a steam inhalation which helps to relieve tension and anxiety.

Other benefits from hops include:

- ❖ Their effectiveness when used in aromatherapy to reduce muscle tension, soreness, and stiffness
- ❖ As a general analgesic: hops contain the ability to relieve pain
- ❖ Can improve sexual performance enhancing libido
- ❖ Will help to reduce menstruation and menstruation cramps
- ❖ Can help to repair respiratory infection or ailments
- ❖ When used as part of a hair care treatment, can enhance

A word of caution

1. Always use essential oils in moderation.
2. Use reliable sources when buying.
3. Always seek medical or professional advice before using them for internal use as in cooking or for internal bodily disorders.

Skin care: though using essential oils seems a reliable way to healthy skin, some concentrated oils can cause an allergic reaction. Most oils should be used with care and combined with a carrier oil such as coconut, avocado and olive oil. A carrier oil is derived from the flesh of fruit, nut or seed by cold-pressing.

Ingesting care: essential oils should not be swallowed. Peppermint, spearmint and other oils, though they may be recommended for edible consumption, should only be taken under strict medical and professional advice.

Bibliography:

Heywood V. H. Chant S. R. (Editors) Popular Encyclopaedia of Plants, Published by Press Syndicate of the University of Cambridge, The Pitt Building, Trumpington Street, Cambridge CB2 1RP, United Kingdom

Friedmann T., M. D., A.B.H.M. Attention Deficit and Hyperactivity Disorder (ADHD) http://files.meetup.com/1481956/ADHD%20Research%20by%20Dr.%20Terry%20 Friedmann.pdf

References

Thank you to the people, and other information collected throughout the years of research for this book.

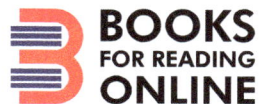

Books That Make A Difference

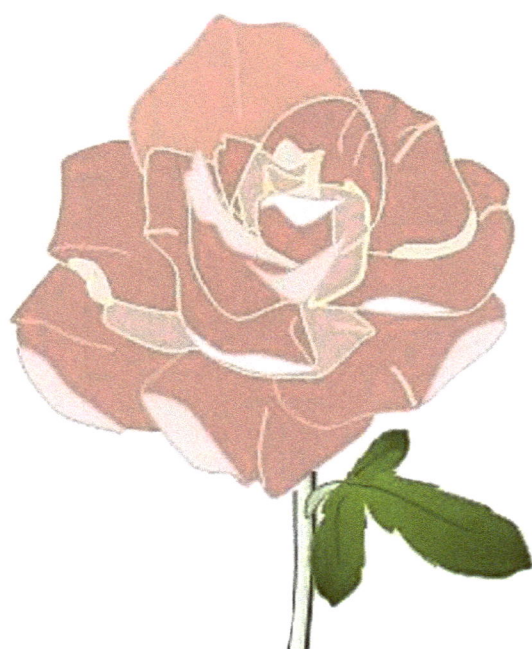

www.ingramcontent.com/pod-product-compliance
Lightning Source LLC
Chambersburg PA
CBHW041101050426
42334CB00063B/3277